Healing Practices
in the South Pacific

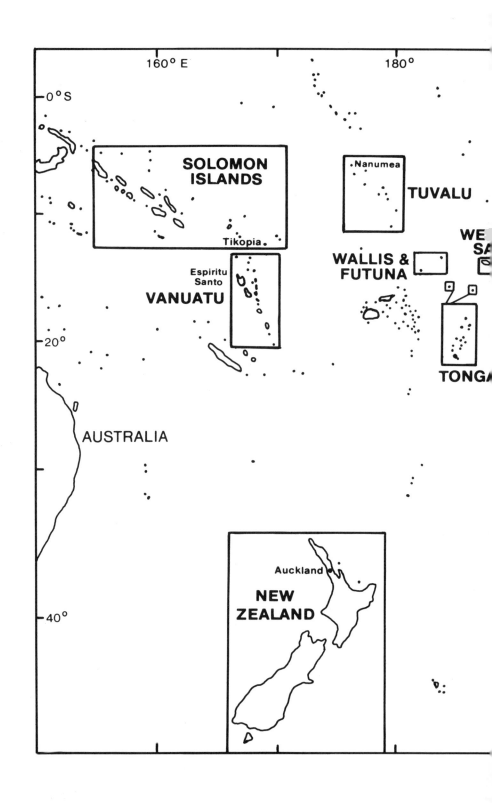

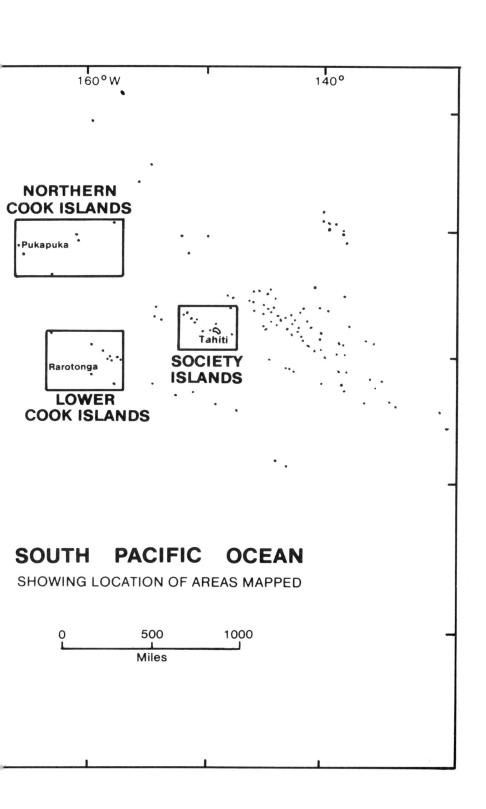

Healing Practices
in the South Pacific

edited by
CLAIRE D. F. PARSONS

PUBLISHED BY
THE INSTITUTE FOR POLYNESIAN STUDIES
BRIGHAM YOUNG UNIVERSITY—HAWAII CAMPUS
IN ASSOCIATION WITH THE
POLYNESIAN CULTURAL CENTER

Paperback Edition 1995

Copyright © 1985 The Institute for Polynesian Studies

All Rights Reserved

Manufactured in the United States of America

The Library of Congress has catalogued the hardcover edition as follows:

Library of Congress Cataloging in Publication Data
Main entry under title:

Healing practices in the South Pacific.

   Bibliography: p.
   Includes index.
   1. Polynesians—Medicine—Addresses, essays, lectures. 2. Medicine, Primitive—Oceania—Addresses, essays, lectures. 3. Folk medicine—Oceania—Addresses, lectures. 4. Healing—Oceania—Addresses, essays, lectures. 5. Social medicines—Oceania—Addresses, essays, lectures. I. Parsons, Claire D. F.
GN670.H43   1985   615.8'82'099   85–14191
ISBN 0–939154–41–2
ISBN 0–939154–56–0 (pbk)

Distributed for The Institute for Polynesian Studies
by the University of Hawai'i Press:

Order Department
University of Hawai'i Press
2840 Kolowalu Street
Honolulu, Hawaii 96822

This book is printed on acid-free paper

Cover art by Barbara McHugh

Contents

Maps		viii
Preface		ix
Acknowledgements		xiii
1	**Samoan Medicine** *Cluny Macpherson*	1
2	**Illness and Healing in Nanumea, Tuvalu** *Anne Chambers and Keith S. Chambers*	16
3	**Healing in Central Espiritu Santo, Vanuatu** *Tomas Ludvigson*	51
4	**Contemporary Healing Practices in Tikopia, Solomon Islands** *Judith Macdonald*	65
5	**Tongan Healing Practices** *Claire D. F. Parsons*	87
6	**Contemporary Healing Practices in East Futuna** *Bruce Biggs*	108
7	**Traditional Healing Practices of Rarotonga, Cook Islands** *Josephine Baddeley*	129
8	**Physical and Social Boundaries in Pukapukan Theories of Disease** *Julia A. Hecht*	144
9	**Tahitian Healing** *Antony Hooper*	158
10	**Midwives and Midwifery in Western Samoa** *Patricia J. Kinloch*	199

11	**Notes on Maori Sickness Knowledge and Healing Practices** Claire D. F. Parsons	213
References		235
Index		245
Contributors		249

Maps

1	*Tuvalu (inset: Nanumea)*	18
2	*Vanuatu*	52
3	*Solomon Islands (inset: Tikopia)*	66
4	*Tonga*	88
5	*Wallis and Futuna*	109
6	*Lower Cook Islands (inset: Rarotonga)*	130
7	*Northern Cook Islands (inset: Pukapuka)*	145
8	*Society Islands*	160
9	*Western Samoa*	200
10	*New Zealand*	214

Maps compiled by Lee S. Motteler
Drawn by Emic Graphics

Preface

During the 1970s worldwide interest developed in traditional healing practices. In 1978 the World Health Organization held a conference on "Traditional Medicine," which concluded by acknowledging the considerable contribution traditional medicine has to offer in the management of sickness. Traditional healing practices, in general, were brought out of disrepute and acknowledged as credible and effective by W.H.O. members. The conference recognized that because research had thus far been "heavily oriented toward medicinal plants, a misleading impression had been given that plant medicines were the only contribution traditional healers could offer health care." The new attitude is revealed in the following statements, contained in the conference proceedings:

> The traditional system of medicine in Sri Lanka meets the basic health needs (physical, emotional, mental, spiritual) of about 70% of the population.
>
> Traditional medicine presents several valuable solutions to the management of culturally-linked diseases and other health problems, and the reason for this spectacular success is that it is an integral part of the people's culture and they have a deep confidence in it.
>
> W.H.O. recognises traditional medicine's effectiveness in control of alcoholism, rheumatoid arthritis, cardiovascular disease, burns, acute abdominal ailments, bone fractures, kidney stones and gall stones.

Having recognized the effectiveness of other practices, western health professionals are now attempting to integrate these systems of knowledge.

Almost inevitably, when confronted by an array of sicknesses and therapies, questions are raised as to their logic, rationality, validity, and effectiveness. As this book shows, western science is not the only form of logic, or rationality, available to mankind. Western medicine cannot justifiably be used as the yardstick against which all other healing practices *must* measure their effectiveness. Who do we ask, the scientist or the patient, for proof of the effectiveness of a "cure"? Who do we ask if acupuncture is effective? Or whether the patient still has chest pain after therapy has been given? This dilemma always leaves room for alternative explanations and treatments of sickness.

If we use science as our epistemology and therefore our criterion for evaluation, we will search for scientific evidence to demonstrate the effectiveness of such practices. However, the whole phenomenon of defining and managing sickness is more complex than this, and the social scientist usually refrains from making such judgments, instead asking questions as to the meaning of each practice for the people concerned. There is an inevitable conflict here for social scientists, and any value judgments implicit in their studies tend to polarize into a pro-science or anti-science polemic. The conflicts of interpretation arising about research into indigenous healing practices are the same conflicts that arise in the clinical situation where competing explanatory models of sickness and therapy engender "problems" in clinical management, communication, and "patient satisfaction." Such conflicts influence psychosocial and biophysical responses in the individual.

This book is primarily written for the Pacific Island people, but it is also addressed to western health professionals, to those interested in medical social science, and to other students of cross-cultural studies. For those interested in health education and in the cost of health care, a culture-sensitive approach would increase efficiency. That is, primary and secondary health care can become more effective if the health professional begins any communication by discussing what is important to the recipient, using sickness concepts relevant to their worldview. Health education programs that are culture-sensitive must inevitably prove to be more sound theoretically. Any educational program can only be as effective as the quality of knowledge that goes into designing it. Poor quality input results in poor quality output. This is costly, time consuming, and of little value to either participant.

While this book presents mainly descriptive research, the acknowledged task of medical social science is to build an interdisciplinary bridge between the biomedical sciences and the sociocultural sciences. This book raises questions about such a relationship in the South Pacific basin specifically, although there are ramifications for other cultural groups. The dialectic is presented between western and Polynesian approaches to healing the sick in terms of the contemporary structure and function of indigenous healing practices, pluralism, and prospective social change. This book is not just of academic or theoretical interest, but of practical relevance in terms of possible constructive directions for the health professional who is willing to accommodate the sickness explanations of individual Pacific Island groups.

It may be noted that a "pattern" of similarity in practices and beliefs emerges among the South Pacific peoples (and such patterns may be useful for the reader to gain a general impression of trends), but it is the personal idiosyncrasies which become important in the day-to-day care of sick people. It is the individual's sickness interpretations that arise in actual sickness situations and it is these "sickness realities" which will assist or confound the management of that instance of sickness.

Readers seeking generalizations that "all" Maoris or "all" Samoans think this or do that will become aware that it is not possible to "neaten up," or generalize, in such a way. There is a great deal of variation between belief and practice in the everyday world. This variation shows the actual processive development and the flexibility and adaptability involved in social change. Hence, among South Pacific peoples there are differences within a group, between tribes, and between urban and rural dwellers.

Throughout this book, a variety of comparisons can be made, region by region, intraculturally and interculturally. Cross-cultural comparisons can be made at the level of diagnosis, sickness explanatory models, and therapy. These descriptions of contemporary healing practices in the Pacific prepare the ground for further research. Indeed, while detailed analyses were not appropriate to a book of this type, some of the contributors have already extended their research and subjected their findings to more extensive analyses. It should become evident that such indigenous healing practices are not simply a matter of a handful of herbs and a headful of superstitions, old traditions lingering on as redundant, ineffective practices. Rather, they should be seen, for the most part, as being adaptive and relevant to contemporary living.

In the past, westerners have assumed that indigenous medical practices had become increasingly redundant with the introduction of western medicine. However, it has been shown that they have, in fact, developed concurrently with the introduction of western medicine. Indeed, in a number of instances, healing practices continue to develop and will not readily be displaced by western medicine. This is in part due to the fact that, in spite of the western view of traditional medicine, the people themselves usually look to their own practices as being complementary to, and not in competition with, western medicine.

Works on the Tokelau Islands, Fiji, Niue, and New Guinea have been omitted for particular reasons. Professor Antony Hooper and Dr. Judith Huntsman, who have been involved in a long-term study in the Tokelau Islands, believe that there are few, if any, indigenous healing practices in the Tokelaus as western medicine has wholly supplanted the traditional practices. Dr. Maçu Salato is currently engaged in studies in ethnomedicine in Fiji but felt it premature to publish any information. This was also true of current research in Niue. New Guinea has been relatively widely studied and a number of works are already available, including papers from the 1982 conference, "Sorcery, Healing and Magic in Melanesia," at La Trobe University, Melbourne, Australia.

Contributions to the book were sought initially from members of each cultural group. However, for a number of reasons, these contributions were not forthcoming. It is hoped that they will become available in the future. The chapter on Maori healing practices, originally to be written by a member of the Maori community, likewise did not materialize; at the last moment it became necessary to draw on my own notes from various Maori individuals and groups. The chapter reflects these opinions rather than detailed research.

In spite of these factors, the book which has emerged presents the majority of the Polynesian peoples' responses to sickness. The contributors are members of different theoretical and methodological persuasions in sociology and anthropology. In the editing of the book, I have tried to keep the potential reader in mind, attempting a balance between consistency of theme and the academic integrity of the authors' works. The reader will find a variety of styles and approaches to the central theme of contemporary healing practices among the Pacific people. The chapters have been arranged in order of the relative emphasis that each assigns to diagnosis, sickness explanation in general, and therapy.

This book is the first collection of studies on contemporary healing practices in the South Pacific. It encompasses more than ethnomedicine as it includes all phases of the sickness process requiring both knowledge and practice—hence the use of the term "healing practices" to include this total spectrum of responses to the phenomenon of sickness.

CLAIRE D. F. PARSONS
October 1984

Acknowledgements

I wish to thank the contributors to this book and the funding agencies that made it possible for the contributors to conduct their research. I also wish to specially acknowledge the people of the South Pacific who patiently assisted the researchers in their efforts to understand their individual sickness realities.

My personal thanks go to Mrs. Sharon Harris, who retyped my own drafts under pressure of deadlines, and to others who assisted in the production of this book.

1

Samoan Medicine

Cluny Macpherson

There is in Western Samoa a body of belief and practice relating to health and illness which is widely believed to be indigenous. It exists alongside an introduced body of belief and practice and together the systems provide the Samoans with health care. The success of the older medical system deserves comment because elsewhere the pressure exerted by introduced systems has led to the decline of indigenous ones. In this account of the development and practice of Samoan medicine I focus on the factors which have contributed to its persistence and show that the contact occurring since 1830 has provided both motive and opportunity for an expansion of the indigenous medical system, and not, as has happened elsewhere, the conditions for its displacement or decline. This process can be seen in several areas: an expansion of beliefs about illness and health; an expansion of the range of therapies used in the management of illness; and an increased range of personnel involved in therapy. Evidence for expansion comes from a comparison of accounts recorded by early and competent visitors to the Samoas[1] with observations of contemporary practice. I also show that in this expansion the indigenous system has incorporated beliefs and practices which have improved its effectiveness. Contemporary Samoan medicine, although regarded as indigenous by its users, is in fact a composite body of belief and practice.

THE PRECONTACT PARADIGM

Most medical paradigms have two elements: a series of beliefs about the nature of health and illness, and a related series of beliefs about appropriate forms of intervention. Since the way in which people conceive of illness determines their response to it, changes in belief generally precede changes in practice. It is to this history that I now turn.

For a very considerable time, Samoan beliefs about illness and strategies of intervention remained relatively stable. All serious illnesses and many less serious ones were thought to be produced by supernatural agents of various types known by the generic term *aitu*. Illness was thought to be an indication of an *aitu*'s displeasure with human behavior, and this belief led victims of illness and their associates to review their behavior to identify actions which might have given offense to the *aitu*. Identification of offender and offense made possible the execution of an appropriate intervention, usually focusing on appeasement of an *aitu*. If the procedure was carried out correctly, the *aitu* removed the sign of its displeasure and the community was free to resume daily life until such time as further offense was given. If the procedure was not carried out correctly, the sick person became progressively more ill and eventually death could occur.

Since symptoms in this model were regarded as indications of displeasure on the part of the *aitu*, the attention that was focused on the symptoms sought clues to the nature of the offense rather than indications of the state of the organism. There was no reason to suppose that biological agents per se were associated with the onset of illness and therefore no reason to suppose that some form of biological intervention would be effective. It is not surprising in such circumstances that a biological model of illness did not emerge. The paradigm was structured in such a way as to explain virtually any outcome of illness, and there was no reason to doubt its adequacy or seek to expand it.

Paradigms tend to be most successful when the number of variables which they must include and the range of outcomes which they must explain are limited. In Samoa before 1830, the range of illnesses which the medical paradigm had to explain was limited by minimal contact with the outside world and by beliefs and practices which reduced the risk of environmental illnesses.[2] Enjoying their geographical isolation, the Samoans showed a marked reluctance to encourage visits by outsiders, apparently stemming from an occasion in which the arrival of visitors had coincided with the onset of a previously unknown disease—possibly cholera, according to Turner—for which they were subsequently held responsible. The disease must have been serious because, at contact, the Samoans were still offering regular prayers to discourage further visits by the "sailing gods." Although contact with Europeans began in 1722, when the Dutch navigator Roggewein sighted the Samoas and recorded their existence, it did not gain momentum for some time because of an incident involving the French navigator La Pérouse, which earned the Samoans a reputation, probably undeserved, for hostility. In the circumstances, the likelihood of the introduction of new diseases or new paradigms was limited. The isolation, however, was not to continue indefinitely.

CONTACT AND DILEMMA

In 1830 John Williams of the London Missionary Society arrived at Sapapali'i, in Savai'i, with a small party of teachers and a Samoan *matai*, Faueā, whom they had taken on board in Tonga. The party was ill on arrival with influenza and, in a remarkable demonstration of poor judgment, Williams allowed the Samoan villagers to take the entire party ashore to allow them to rest at two different villages. Williams's own journal records that the party was very ill and at least one died during the stay. This episode was only the first of a number of visits which introduced new diseases to the Samoas, effectively ending the period of epidemiological stability. Between 1830 and 1918 the record is dismal, for among the diseases introduced were several which resulted in epidemics that successively devastated various sections of the Samoan population.

The Samoans had in effect two options: to abandon the precontact medical paradigm, which by now was proving inadequate to explain the new diseases, or to extend it to provide explanations of the new range and types of illness. That they chose the latter course requires some explanation. First, the illnesses which their own paradigm had explained so well continued to afflict Samoans, and there was no reason to suppose that the *aitu* who had dominated their lives for so long had suddenly relinquished their power. Even the Samoans who were converted to Christianity did not, to the missionaries' despair, abandon their belief in the power of the *aitu*. The role of supernatural agents in sickness, then, was not denied. It is acknowledged today. But this belief could not, on its own, explain new patterns of illness.

Secondly, the missionaries and other Europeans were not particularly successful in preventing or treating the illnesses among their own ranks. The mission record is a depressing one involving a remarkable number of deaths, miscarriages, protracted illnesses, and departures from the field on account of sickness. This vulnerability was due to limited medical expertise and also to the fact that many arrived unaccustomed to the climate and living conditions which they found in Samoa. Since only a few missionaries were medically qualified, most were obliged to fall back on prayer and a small range of herbs and simples in cases of illness. The tragic record of the missions can hardly have impressed the Samoans with the superiority of the medical practice which the visitors introduced; in many respects, they suffered worse health than the Samoans. Moreover, the medicine available in the missions was crude and certainly not typical of western medical practice at the time. The Samoans had, for practical purposes, only the missionary practice on which to base their evaluation of the introduced medical paradigm, and could have been forgiven for a somewhat pessimistic evaluation of its potential.[3] Thus the

Samoans found themselves in a situation which demanded new ways of thinking about and responding to new illnesses which their precontact paradigm alone could not provide. As the need was becoming apparent, so too were the means for expansion becoming readily available, and it is to this process which we now turn.

EXPANSION OF THE PARADIGM

In a situation which demanded new responses to illness, the Samoans had opportunity to borrow from the missionaries those practices which seemed to be effective in the management of illness. The missionaries' experimentation with local flora had not gone unnoticed and in some cases had led to the discovery of herbal remedies which were then made available to Samoan parishioners. Certain of these remedies were said to be more effective than the Samoan practices current at the time, and there is evidence that the Samoans seized with some enthusiasm the possibility of experimenting with plant material. In addition, the missions made available surgical skills which extended knowledge of the possibilities of this form of intervention. But perhaps the most important result of contact with the missionaries was the realization that although the missionaries had access to an omnipotent deity, their explanations of illness and their strategies of intervention in many cases accorded only a minimal role to that deity. Thus the missionaries introduced the possibility of simultaneous belief in the omnipotence of a deity and a greater human role in the management of illness.

Other sources of new information were gradually becoming available. By 1866 the missionary Thomas Powell had translated into Samoan a zoology manual which contained, among other things, an extensive discussion of human anatomy and physiology; the manual was intended for graduate pastors who were unfamiliar with concepts which they would find necessary in their teaching. Also notable was a manual of public health which was written and translated into Samoan in 1902, in an attempt by the U. S. Naval administration in Pago Pago to raise the standard of public health. These manuals, and others, contained a wealth of information in a coherent and readable form, and they were made available at a time when Samoans were seeking new information about illness and its management.

Additional sources of information were also becoming available. Samoan pastors who had been trained at the Malua Theological Seminary and sent to islands in Western Polynesia and Melanesia returned to Samoa with medical beliefs and practices from those islands. There are plants in use in Samoa today which are known to be exotic, and cures which are known to have been brought from Papua New Guinea, where many pastors have served. Other Samoans were recruited as crew for ships operating in the region and traveled throughout the Pacific. These ships visited Samoa regularly and sometimes left non-Samoan crewmen behind. Many of the Tongans and Hawaiians, whom Turner and others note as the most skilled native healers in Samoa at the time, found their way to Samoa by this means.

Then, around the turn of the century, significant numbers of Melanesians and Chinese were brought to Samoa to work on the plantations. Although it was believed that contact between the indentured labor and the Samoan population should be limited as far as possible, attempts to do this were far less successful than their European sponsors had hoped. There were numerous interracial unions, which were later formalized, and today there is a substantial part-Chinese, and a somewhat smaller part-Melanesian, population in Samoa. This admixture probably also contributed to the borrowing of medical information from non-Samoan sources. The conclusion of international agreements in 1899 vested control of what is now Western Samoa in German hands and what is now American Samoa in the hands of the United States. Each of the administrations embarked on campaigns to raise standards of health in their respective territories. This period saw increasing numbers of Samoans become involved in the public health programs. Their involvement brought them into close contact with introduced beliefs and practices and provided further opportunities for borrowing and incorporation of these ideas in the "indigenous" system. Samoan medical professionals, for example, would sometimes modify traditional practices by introducing new substances into the repertoire, in the belief that this would make more effective that which could not be changed (Keesing 1934, 397ff.). And attempts were made to extend health care into the villages, with interesting consequences. These programs sought as trainees people with status who were trusted in their villages. Often those who were nominated for training as village-level workers were people already working as traditional healers. At the conclusion of their training they were provided with equipment and a variety of drugs and returned to their villages. It is uncertain whether those who obtained treatment from these health workers were at all aware of the origins of their cure, whether indigenous or introduced, since they were naturally more concerned with its effectiveness. There were undoubtedly situations where patients assumed that because a treatment was dispensed by a *fofo* or "healer," it was an indigenous cure, whether or not that was actually the case.

The transmission of treatments without accounts of their origins, or of the logic which underpins them, has continued to the present, and has become even more complicated by a recent trend reported by healers. They state that some of their less scrupulous patients have observed the preparation and administration of treatments and have then attempted to replicate the cure without the consent of the healer—in some cases with a measure of success.[4] These healers wonder whether such a process might not have been occurring for rather longer than they had suspected. The result of this process is the incorporation of treatments about which little is known, since the circumstances in which they were acquired prevent disclosure of their origin.

All of this, of course, further confuses any attempt to establish the origins of healers' repertoires. We must simply accept the fact that the so-called indigenous medical system is an augmented one which is held by its users to be indigenous not because of its actual origins, but because of its relationship to the introduced system. In other words, it is indigenous because it is Samoan rather than western, and as such it is associated with a different etiology which underpins a different set of practices.

Whereas the precontact paradigm assigned a central role, in both causation and treatment, to various supernatural agencies, the augmented indigenous paradigm includes a wider range of causal possibilities and in turn allows for a wider range of treatments. There is no reason to suppose that this process of expansion has stopped, for the reasons outlined above, or that further expansion is impossible.

INDIGENOUS AND INTRODUCED PARADIGMS

The arrival of Europeans and of diseases previously unknown in Samoa led to the expansion of the indigenous paradigm which has been outlined above. The augmented system that resulted could not, however, incorporate certain features of the postcontact situation, such as epidemic illnesses, and these illnesses and their treatment were understood to belong to the introduced system.[5] Many Samoans believe that *ma'i palagi,* illnesses of European origin, are, like their own illnesses, *ma'i samoa,* most effectively treated by those who have had experience of them. Healers point out that European medicine cannot treat many Samoan illnesses successfully because it does not acknowledge the existence of certain elements necessary to effective diagnosis and treatment. Similarly, they believe that Samoan healers cannot treat many European illnesses because they do not have access to the necessary information about those illnesses.

The paradigms are thus seen not as competing systems, but as more or less complementary ones. This belief is sustained by evidence of the advantages of cooperation. Healers presented with cases of *ma'i palagi* can refer these patients to practitioners of European medicine for treatment, and doctors trained in European medicine can similarly refer patients with a Samoan illness to a healer. It is easy, however, to exaggerate the neatness of the boundaries between the two systems. In practice, it is often difficult to identify the "real" nature of any given illness and to decide what is the most appropriate treatment. Some practitioners of European medicine are less willing to refer patients to Samoan healers than others, and the same can be said of Samoan practitioners. Some patients insist on taking treatments from the two systems simultaneously, especially if there is doubt about the diagnosis, such as when an illness fails to follow the expected course.

Despite these difficulties, Samoans do not regard the two systems as mutually exclusive. Indeed, many move between them without any sense of inconsistency. This seems to be possible for several reasons. First, although there are important differences in belief between the two systems concerning such matters as anatomy, physiology, and psychiatry, these differences are not necessarily apparent to practitioners and their patients. Only rarely would such contradictions come into view.[6] Since the users see practitioners in both systems referring patients between the two, they have no reason to believe that there is any serious inconsistency. Healers observe that if they did not in fact believe that European medicine was effective they would not refer people to its practitioners, and they presumed that the same reasoning was behind the European-trained practitioners' decisions to refer their patients to Samoan practitioners. If those who are in a position to understand the systems act as if there are no inconsistencies, there is no good reason for less well informed users to suspect that there are. Furthermore, since patients can take treatments from both systems simultaneously, or serially, it is often difficult for them to establish which treatment was successful in any given case. The tendency is to avoid judgment, or rejection of one for the other, by simply resolving to take the two treatments simultaneously should future circumstances warrant it. Thus, while less than perfect in practice, a form of integration between the two systems does exist which provides the basis for a stable coexistence.

Samoan medicine has evolved from a system in which a practitioner had only to decide which supernatural agency was involved to one in which an expanded range of causal agencies is acknowledged.[7] While supernatural agents remain a significant feature of the etiology of Samoan illnesses, they have been displaced as the primary cause, a fact which has undoubtedly enhanced the system's explanatory power and effectiveness. I turn now to an examination of the role of healers in Samoan medicine and how that role has changed since contact.

HEALERS AND THEIR ROLE IN SAMOAN MEDICINE

First, as a frame of reference, we consider briefly the role of healers in precontact Samoa. J. B. Stair noted that the Samoan priesthood, the *taula-aitu* or "anchors of the spirits," could be divided into four classes.

One class was principally involved in the treatment of illness. These *taula-aitu-o-āiga* or "priests of families" were, according to Stair, mediums who communicated with the family gods, and the office was usually held by a family member. Stair does not indicate whether the class was restricted to particular families and says only that "it was sometimes held by the head of the family or his sister." This priest would summon the family gods and seek their assistance in "effecting the recovery of some sick person placed before him" (Stair 1897, 222). The family god, through the priest, conveyed instructions for the management of the illness, which the family obeyed. Missionary accounts of this procedure are somewhat skeptical of its value, noting that the principal beneficiaries were the family priests themselves, who enjoyed the fame which accompanied successful treatments and accepted the gifts made to the god on whose behalf they acted. Furthermore, as Stair points out, failure to cure an illness was not taken as evidence of their inadequacy but rather as an indication of the superiority of other hostile gods, and so their own power was, in effect, unquestioned.

A second class of the priesthood was occasionally involved in the treatment of illness. They were known as the *taula-aitu-vavalo-ma-fai-tuʻi* or "anchors of the spirits to predict and curse." These priests or sorcerers communicated with gods who in turn revealed the identities of people who had caused some form of misfortune to another. When illness was suspected to have been the result of a curse, a priest of this type was asked to identify the cursor, the cause of the curse, and the appropriate form of placation. The missionaries were equally skeptical about these priests, who were similarly immune to exposure and received "large presents of food and valuable property" for their services (Stair 1897, 225).

There were also healers not connected with the priesthood who applied various forms of massage and used herbal medicines. This group, known as *fo-maʻi*, did not play a significant role in the treatment of illness. They seem to have specialized in two kinds of massage, *milimili* and *lomilomi,* for headaches and muscular pains respectively, and also experimented less successfully with herbs and simples. In a summary of the state of the Samoan medical arts, Stair notes: "Although they had much sickness their remedies were few, and for the most part unreliable notwithstanding the fact that the flora of the group included many medicinal plants and herbs of much value" (1897, 164).

Missionary accounts of Samoan medicine tend to dwell on the more spectacular or otherworldly dimensions of the practices they encountered, and their evident interest in the role of the various priests may have led them to understate the importance of other kinds of healers in the treatment of illness. Yet nonmissionary accounts also support the conclusion that it was the *taula-aitu* who traditionally played the central role in treating illness, with other healers serving less important functions. In contemporary Samoan medicine, by contrast, a rather more diverse range of personnel and approaches to healing is evident.

Most Samoan adults could be considered healers of a sort because they have some knowledge of common illnesses and remedies. As Schoeffel notes, most have knowledge of the commonly used medicinal plants and are able to prepare treatments with them (1980, 390). This "first aid kit" is also likely to include a few introduced practices, such as the use of aspirin and epsom salts. These adults do not refer to themselves as healers or *fofo*, however; they confine their efforts to minor common illnesses and are usually quite willing to pass on problems to specialists as soon as they can.

The specialists to whom such cases are referred are known by the generic term *fofo* 'healer'. *Fofo* are people with varying amounts of knowledge and levels of skill. The most useful distinction is between *taulasea* and *taula-aitu*, based on the former's skill in the treatment of *ma'i samoa* 'Samoan illness' and the latter's skill in the treatment of *ma'i aitu* 'ghost illness', which is believed to involve supernatural agency. These categories are not exclusive and some healers practice both as *taulasea* and as *taula-aitu*, treating all types of Samoan illness. Although available in formal speech, the distinction between the two kinds of healer is not normally made in everyday speech, where the term *fofo* is used and qualified only when necessary. The distinction between the two is elaborated here in the interest of clarity.

Taulasea treat illnesses which are beyond the range of first aid but do not seem to involve supernatural agency. As healers they are thought to have esoteric knowledge which permits them to understand illness, and typically they are very religious people who believe that such powers or talents as they may possess are gifts of God. In this respect they regard themselves as those to whom the Lord has chosen to impart the gift of healing referred to in scripture. Some believe that their knowledge is insufficient on its own to ensure a cure and that the success of the cure is dependent on maintaining their relationship with God. Others, while admitting a connection between the efficacy of the cure and their relationship with God, contend that since possession of their knowledge predated commitment to Christianity, their power does not derive directly from it but is sanctioned by God because the practice of healing is in accord with Christian principles.

The role is not clearly related to gender: while there do seem to be correlations between types of practice and gender, these seem to be coincidental products of the traditional division of labor. Healers explained the apparent correlation as coincidence, noting, in some cases, that God was free to bestow the gift of healing on whomsoever he pleased and they could not be expected to explain God's choice.[8]

A *taulasea*'s medical knowledge is typically learned in adolescence and early adulthood, and it is usually obtained from a single source. The repertoire is then supplemented with cures from other healers, possibly from grateful patients, and from experimentation. A healer's knowledge is usually, but not necessarily, passed on to a kinsperson. The person to whom the knowledge is transmitted must be someone of good character[9] who has demonstrated both a desire to learn and an aptitude for medicine. An interesting consequence of the first requirement is that the knowledge tends to be placed in the hands of people who are conspicuously Christian, which undoubtedly helps to remove whatever stigma may be associated with its pre-Christian origins.

An apprentice's training is gained by watching the healer at work as time permits. *Fofo* apparently have nothing like the *whare wananga* of the Maori, to which students were sent for long periods of time to acquire esoteric knowledge. Some knowledge is acquired incidentally by healers' children who collect the ingredients for medicine, are present as the healer works, and accompany the healers on visits to patients. More formal instruction is given during the practice of medicine, although some knowledge, because of its more esoteric nature, is given privately after patients have gone. The amount of knowledge transmitted during the training depends on the interaction between healer and learner and their respective capabilities. While their relationship is clearly a deferential one, it does not seem to be characterized by extreme deference and does not involve explicit rights and obligations which are binding on either party.

Healers receive gifts *(mea'alofa)* for their services but do not ask for them; they strenuously resist the suggestion that gifts are in fact payment for services. In some cases, healers will attempt to persuade the patient to take back all or part of the gift or will suggest that, since the treatment is God's work, the patient make a gift to the church instead. This reluctance to accept gifts is based on the belief that God-given talents can be taken away if they are abused. Most healers will accept small gifts and fares where travel is involved; to refuse would be discourteous, they say, since it would imply that they believed the donor's family to be too poor to afford such gifts.[10] There is no obligation on the patient to make such a gift, and no expectation of a gift in cases where the treatment is unsuccessful. It seems that the more significant aspect of the healer's reward is the deference which he or she receives from patients and their associates.

Healers who deal with physical illness are of two kinds. The first, known as *fogau*, treat breaks and tears such as bone fractures, dislocations, muscular pains, and sprains. Although usually male, being so is not required by tradition, and indeed there are female *fogau*. The second, known as *taulasea* proper, treat skin and internal illnesses. They are usually female, but again there are male *taulasea*. The categories are not exclusive and there are individuals who practice both skills.

The *fogau*'s treatment of pain in the muscles or joints is one of the oldest forms of Samoan medicine; it is among those which were reported by the earliest missionaries. Diagnosis takes place through a process of questioning and probing. The questions typically focus on the activities and events preceding the onset of pain. The treatment usually involves one or more of the following: massage, manipulation, cold compresses, immobilization of the injury, and splinting of suspected fractures. In most cases, *fogau* have an idea of the time it will take to treat the injury; if the injury fails to respond in that time, the *fogau* will revise the initial diagnosis by paying attention to the state of the symptoms, such as bruising, supplemented by the patient's report on the condition. The pattern of treatment is determined as it proceeds, and there is nothing which could be considered ritualistic about it. Apart from the actual physical treatment, the *fogau* will give advice about activities which the patient should avoid and instructions about symptoms which the patient must report. If the *fogau* decides that the patient's condition is beyond his skill, the patient may be referred either to another *fogau* or to the hospital for further treatment. The patient is likewise free to seek another *fogau*'s services if progress has been unsatisfactory or if there is doubt about the accuracy of the diagnosis. *Fogau* are an important part of the indigenous medical practice and their services are widely sought and held by Samoans to be effective.

Taulasea treat external and internal illnesses, and as a group they include practitioners with varying degrees of specialization. Some treat a wide range of illnesses and will accept most patients who present themselves. Others tend to specialize in several types of illness while others specialize still further, confining their practice to a particular illness; in both cases they may refuse to treat others. As healers become recognized for their skill with particular illnesses their practice tends increasingly to focus on those illnesses, and in these cases some sort of de facto specialization occurs. Those who specialize do recognize other symptoms, however, and can refer patients to the appropriate healer. Healers are thus known by their skills, which may be associated with particular illnesses, parts of the body, age groups, or to a lesser extent gender. Their services are normally sought by patients with illnesses for which they are thought to have a cure.

The *taulasea* begins by establishing that the symptoms do indicate a physical and not a supernatural illness and then, having identified the illness, initiates the treatment. The treatment can involve massage and manipulation, the manufacture and administration of herbal medicines, the use of various forms of poultice, enema, emetic, inhalation, and dressing. In some cases it can include minor surgical procedures. The treatment continues until the condition improves or it becomes clear that a new diagnosis is required. This point is reached when the course of treatment indicated by the initial diagnosis fails to have the predicted effect, or when unexpected symptoms appear. This may suggest that the initial diagnosis was either incorrect or only partially correct and that, in the latter case, a combination of illnesses is involved and treatment must be adjusted to cope with the several illnesses which produced the symptoms.

If after such adjustments the treatment is still without effect, another possibility must be considered. The illness might be one involving supernatural agency. At this point the *taulasea* must decide whether referral is necessary. Some can invoke a new range of skills to become *taula-aitu;* others will decide that the skills required are beyond them and will refer the patient to a *taula-aitu*. In either case a new range of diagnostic skills and treatments is called for.

The *taula-aitu* must first establish what *aitu* is involved and the nature of the event giving rise to the *aitu*'s annoyance. If it is one of the major *aitu,* known as Nifoloa, Sauma'iafe, and Telesa (Goodman 1971), a course of action will be followed which aims at discovering the nature of the offense and arriving at some form of conciliation. The procedure involves the sick person and sometimes his or her associates, who will review their behavior in the period preceding the onset of the illness. The treatment may also include simultaneous intercession by the *taula-aitu* and administration of physical remedies, and it can vary from one *taula-aitu* to another.

If the *taula-aitu* decides that none of the major *aitu* is involved, attention will then focus on the family *aitu*. In some cases these family *aitu* are well known through previous manifestations; in other cases it might be that the *aitu* has never been encountered before. The intervention is usually the consequence of misbehavior which the *aitu* has witnessed, and the patient must identify and admit to it before recovery is possible. This process is aided by application of a fairly well known set of behavioral standards, which when not adhered to can be expected to provoke some form of supernatural intervention. Diagnosis focuses on these areas first. The diagnosis, however, can be complicated by the fact that *aitu* sometimes vent displeasure on a relation of the transgressor, which means that the conduct of the patient's family and friends must also be reviewed in cases where the patient's own conduct does not seem to provide a clue.[11]

The *aitu* who is involved in the illness can reveal the source of its displeasure and the conciliatory gesture that is demanded. This revelation occurs when the patient, apparently in trance, speaks in a voice other than his own to explain the nature of the transgression and the appropriate course of action. The patient's associates usually recognize the voice and its identity is a clue to the seriousness of the problem. Some *aitu* intervene only with good cause, and usually over an event or series of events which reflects unjustly on their reputation or that of their family. Their complaints and demands are taken seriously and when carried out tend to lead to recovery.[12] There are other *aitu* whose complaints are taken less seriously and who are regarded as an annoyance. When dealing with these *aitu*, the patient and his associates may decide that no conciliatory gesture is appropriate, or indeed that such a gesture has already been made; a decision will then be made to attempt some form of retaliation against the *aitu* (Goodman 1971; Shore 1977).

Throughout the process of diagnosis the *taula-aitu* can continue to administer physical remedies believed to be effective in the treatment of ghost sickness. These medicines are known as *vai aitu* and their composition is usually a well-kept secret. The role which they play in the recovery is unclear. Since some of the plants used are known to have hypotensive properties, it seems likely that they play a more important role than might be supposed. The onset of a ghost sickness, then, does not normally signal suspension of biological intervention but rather indicates a new role for it. It may be that the cures depend on both psychological and biological elements.

CONCLUSION

At the center of the indigenous paradigm is a belief that the normal human condition is one of equilibrium, proof of which can be found in the social environment in which the body functions, and in the body itself. This stability is fragile, and it is regularly disrupted. When disruption occurs the cause must be located and removed, so that balance is restored.

In most illnesses the search for causes begins in the body itself. *Fogau* seek fractured limbs, displaced joints, sprained muscles. *Taulasea* seek displaced or malfunctioning organs and try to restore their normal function. *Taula-aitu* seek supernatural causes of physical malfunction and resolve the disturbance in such a way that social equilibrium is restored. In both the assumptions underlying it and its social function, Samoan medicine seems rather more like its introduced counterpart than one usually tends to assume.

NOTES

This chapter is an outline of a larger work in progress, based on information from several sources. The historical material comes largely from research in the Pacific Collection of Hamilton Library at the University of Hawaii; the assistance of its curator, Renee Heyum, is gratefully acknowledged. The account of contemporary practice comes from observation and interviews with Samoan healers and their patients; these interviews were conducted in Samoan by my wife, La'avasa, and myself, and many were taped in 1980–81. Observation was formalized, involving protracted sessions watching healers at work and listening to them discussing their work. Interviews with western-trained health professionals were conducted, in most cases in English, in Western Samoa in 1977 and 1980. My most recent period of research was made possible through sabbatical leave granted by the University of Auckland, and their generosity is gratefully acknowledged. This work is for La'avasa, without whose patience and assistance the project would have been impossible.

1. The quality of visitors' accounts varies considerably. Those chosen for these comparisons are those generally held to be the most reliable and accurate of the available sources: J. B. Stair, George Turner, Commodore Wilkes, A. B. Steinberger, and Augustin Kramer.

2. The debate over the range of endemic illness occurs because of the state of medical belief during the period at which they were reported, and because those who provided accounts were often not trained to do so and could, and did, confuse illnesses.

3. There were medically qualified residents in the centers in which European populations were concentrated but their skills, while greater than those of the missionaries, were far less apparent to the Samoans.

4. It was formerly believed that such attempts were destined to fail, because treatments, while they could be passed from person to person, would only work if their owner authorized their use. Thus healers openly prepared and even discussed their medicine with their patients.

5. These illnesses include high and low blood pressure, diabetes, measles, tuberculosis, mumps, poliomyelitis, yellow fever, venereal diseases, and influenza. For the last two mentioned, however, healers believe that there are effective indigenous treatments.

6. An example of contradiction: according to western medicine human bones become more likely to break with age; Samoan medicine holds the reverse to be true. The situations in which members of each system collect and review evidence and confirm the correctness of their beliefs are not normally open to those who would contradict the beliefs or challenge their adequacy.

7. This process of expansion is reflected in the greatly increased range of plants and plant compounds used in the management of illness. Contemporary Samoan medical practice depends heavily on a wide range of indigenous and exotic plant species. This appears to be a postcontact development, a conclusion supported by examination of the record of Samoan plant usages over time. An analysis of early editions of Pratt's much-praised dictionary yields very few plant

Samoan Medicine

usages connected with medicine despite large numbers of nonmedicinal plant usages.

8. This tends to confirm the suspicion that the practice of medicine is of post-contact origin, since other roles which have clear gender requirements are well known and associated with elaborate justifications based on tradition.

9. This is necessary since it is widely believed that God is unlikely to sanction either the practice or the treatments of those who are not deserving. This means that only those whose lives are reasonably free of "sin" are likely to qualify as "trainees." Unsuitable trainees would simply fail as healers.

10. These healers hold in low regard those practitioners—typically itinerants in peri-urban villages—who exploit the gratitude of their patients' families by accepting large gifts. This corruption is not common among village-based practitioners who must live among those whom they treat.

11. Readers interested in the consequences of this belief for social control and a sense of collective responsibility will find them documented in Shore 1977 and Schoeffel 1980.

12. Western diagnosis of these conditions is typically of hysteria which is usually associated with guilt. The public revelation of the guilt and the public acceptance of the necessity of conciliatory gesture may remove the cause of the hysteria.

2

Illness and Healing in Nanumea, Tuvalu

Anne Chambers and Keith S. Chambers

"No," answered the local doctor, "I don't believe in sorcery and supernaturally caused illness. Whenever you look deeper at those sorts of things, they turn out to be diseases you can name."

He paused and looked pensive. I felt we had reached a dead end in our conversation, but, after a moment or two, he went on. "You know, a strange thing happened to me when I was going to medical school in Fiji. I began to have problems with my upper back and it was diagnosed as fibrositis. I had this trouble for eight or nine years and each time I went home to Nanumea I noticed it got worse. I used to get my wife to squeeze my back to lessen the pain. Finally, when I was home, my mother resolved to get help from a traditional practitioner. My wife was in on it too, and one day they told me to come along with them, that they had arranged for me to see this man. I was surprised and a bit angry, but I went. The old man had me sit near a large tub of water with some leaves in it. Then he whirled a red hot axe head around me and put some of the water from the tub on me, by poking with a stick or his finger. He put a wreath of flowers on my head. I was very frightened of the red hot axe. But from that time on, my back problems went away. The old man's assistant told me that someone had done sorcery to me to cause my sore back."

Curing rituals such as this, involving heated axe heads, floral head wreaths, and specially treated coconut oil are as much a part of healing in the atoll community of Nanumea, Tuvalu, as are antibiotics and the diagnostic techniques of western medicine. This chapter describes the variety of healing practices used there and their relationship to each other. It also discusses local theories of the causes of death and illness, the choices made between the available therapies, and some general features of Nanumean healing beliefs.[1] Though western medicine provides assistance for both routine, minor health problems and serious injuries and diseases, Nanumeans also use herbal remedies, massage, pressure application, bloodletting, and heat application to treat their afflictions. In addition, therapeutic rituals provide treatment for and protections against the illnesses caused by sorcery. Because most of our information was collected during field research in Nanumea, we focus explicitly on the healing practices of that community. However, we have also included relevant statistical information for Tuvalu as a whole, as well as ethnographic data for other Tuvalu communities as far as this is available to us. We expect that the healing practices and attitudes we describe for Nanumea are roughly similar to those found elsewhere in Tuvalu.

After briefly outlining the major geographic and social features of Nanumea, we go on to describe the situation within which healing occurs in this community. Mortality rates, economic conditions, sanitation practices, common illnesses, and the impact made by sickness on people's time all play a role in forming the Nanumean health context. We then discuss local ideas about the causes of illness and death before describing traditional and western medical therapy used on the atoll.[2] In the concluding section, some general characteristics of Nanumean healing are presented.

NANUMEA AND TUVALU

Nanumea is the northernmost of the nine atolls and low coral islands that make up the Pacific nation of Tuvalu.[3] These islands lie just west of the International Date Line and spread from 5 degrees to just over 11 degrees south of the equator. Nanumea atoll is about 13 km in overall length and nearly 3 km wide. Most of this area is composed of reef and lagoon, and the land area is just 3.8 square km. Rainfall is generally ample, averaging about 2,718 mm (107 inches), and the atoll lies close enough to the equator to escape the brunt of southern Pacific hurricanes. Except for periods of relatively rare prolonged drought, Nanumea has a stable subsistence base capable of sustaining its large population. In 1973, nearly one thousand of the six thousand people resident in Tuvalu lived on Nanumea. Most households, 121 out of 145, are located in the main village clustered around the community's meeting house and church. There is a much smaller subsidiary village on Lakena islet at the far end of the lagoon which provides its inhabitants with easy access to the taro pits located there and also a respite from the often-intense social life in the main village.

The majority of Nanumeans derive their living from the subsistence economy. Men fish in the ocean off the leeward reef in outrigger canoes and also spear and net fish along the reef flats and in the lagoon. Taro and "atoll taro" *(Cyrtosperma)* are grown in intensively cultivated pits

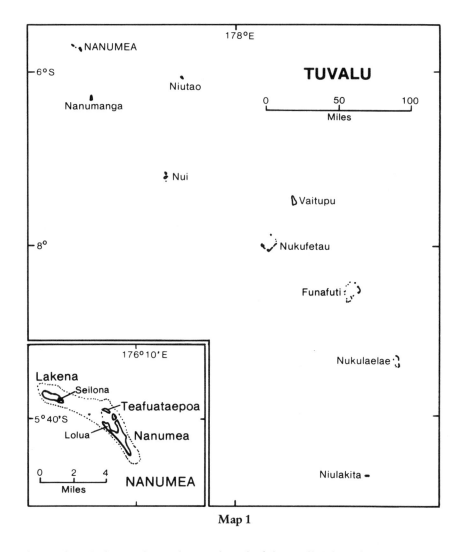

Map 1

located on Lakena islet at the north end of the atoll. The other major traditional food source is the coconut palm, which yields drinking nuts, coconut flesh and its expressed cream, and coconut sap "toddy." Fresh toddy serves as a refreshing and nutritious drink, a mildly sweetening ingredient in cooking, and may be processed through boiling into a long-keeping molasses. (The fresh drink also becomes alcoholic if allowed to ferment.) These locally produced foods form the core of the diet. They are augmented by a variety of imported foods available from the Nanumea branch of the local cooperative society. These include flour, rice, sugar, canned fish and meat, tea and coffee, among other items. Nanumea's vegetation and fauna are those typical of coral atolls.

In precontact times the dispersed islands of Tuvalu shared many cultural and linguistic features in common, though there was also considerable variation among them. The islands were apparently never united into a single political unit until the imposition of British colonial rule in the late nineteenth century, but interisland voyaging contacts were common, and two or three islands joined together in shifting alliances from time to time. Britain declared Tuvalu a protectorate in 1892, by which time there had already been extensive missionary activity by Samoan pastors from the London Missionary Society, and a long history of resident traders representing various Pacific trading concerns (Kofe 1976; Macdonald 1982; Munro 1980; Brady 1975). The protectorate was accorded full colonial status in 1916 when Tuvalu and the Micronesian islands of Kiribati to the north, as well as a number of other scattered islands under British control, were united as the Gilbert and Ellice Islands Colony. During the years of colonial rule Britain maintained only a small number of officers in Tuvalu but managed to make considerable changes in lifestyles. Mission activity had already secured the nominal Christianization of the Tuvalu population by the time of the declaration of the protectorate, and church primary schools existed on all Tuvalu islands from the 1870s until the 1960s, when they were supplemented by government schools. Increasing concern among the Tuvaluans over future domination by the more populous Gilbert Islands led to a separation of the two groups in 1975. In 1978 Tuvalu became an independent nation.[4]

In the wake of missionary activity and the formal imposition of British political control, there were necessarily widespread changes in social and political organization in Nanumea, as in the rest of Tuvalu. One of the first significant changes in response to pressure from both church and government was the shift from a series of small lineage-based residential groups, each probably with its own meeting house and central square *(malae)*, to a single village consisting of neat rows of houses focused around a central church and meeting house. The authority of lineage heads, and of priests in the traditional religion, was undermined as the Samoan pastor assumed increasing power. Nanumean political organization with its balanced tension between hereditary chiefly lineages *(aliki)* and lineages of leading warriors *(toa)* was also seriously shaken when the warriors were deposed under missionary influence, and the chiefs were gradually relegated to figurehead status. Political authority is now vested in an elected island council, and Nanumea, along with each island in Tuvalu, is represented in the national legislature which meets in the capital, Funafuti.

THE NANUMEAN HEALTH CONTEXT

A visitor's first impression of Nanumea atoll is one of beauty and cleanliness. Sunlight sparkles off the deep blue ocean water, glints on the waves tumbled onto the reef, sinks down deep in the turquoise lagoon, reflects from the clear shallows. The sea breeze, with its pure salt tang, tosses the palm fronds overhead and cools the tropically warm air. The tides scour the foreshore and flush out the latrines perched on stilts over the reef. In the village area, tall breadfruit trees shade thatched houses with open sides, clearly suited to the climate. The yards around them are immaculate and the sandy atoll soil shows the broom marks from the sweeping which begins each day. Pigs are penned outside the village, the water cisterns are sealed against debris, the public buildings are well maintained. For all its heat and humidity, the atoll seems generally to be a healthy place to live and its people seem to lead vigorous and happy lives.

Demographic statistics (Macrae 1980) only partially support these impressions. They indicate that the Tuvalu health status is moderately favorable, though far from outstanding. Calculations of childhood mortality for the Polynesian population resident in Tuvalu at the time of the 1973 census showed that 892 per 1,000 children survived to their second birthday. The steady improvement in childhood mortality which began in the mid-sixties continued through the next decade. By 1979, census data indicated that male children were surviving to age two at a rate of 934 per 1,000 live births, female children at a rate of 947. While this appears to represent a significant improvement in just a few years, demographers caution that the figures may be somewhat optimistic, since childhood mortality rates seem unduly low by comparison with adult mortality. It appears likely that children's births have been underreported in the censuses (Macrae 1980). On the other hand, medical personnel believe that improvement in medical services and comprehensive government health programs have lowered childhood mortality rates. These programs include health education, vaccination services, a filariasis eradication campaign, and widely available family planning services. Tuvalu's low fertility (2.8 children per woman) and crude birth rates (23.7 per 1,000 total population), which have held steady throughout the seventies, benefit the health of its citizens not only directly but also indirectly by not overtaxing the country's limited medical facilities. Mortality figures from the 1979 census give an expectation of life at birth of 57 years for males and 60 years for females; longer life expectancies apply, of course, for individuals who survive the first and riskiest year. These statistics from the census reports could, potentially, be augmented by the birth and death records which have been kept on each Tuvalu island since early in this century. Unfortunately, neither these records, nor the statistics kept by the Tuvalu hospital at Funafuti, are judged to be complete enough to allow reliable demographic analysis (Macrae 1980).

Tuvalu mortality rates today are roughly comparable to those of other Pacific Island communities, though they appear to be somewhat less favorable (Macrae 1980, 43, 47). Tuvalu's small population (7,271 in 1979) means, of course, that the total numbers of births and deaths are relatively low. Computing survival rates per thousand births is thus subject to random variation as well as potential sampling error, and such rates may not be wholly reliable for use in comparing the situation in Tuvalu with that in other Pacific countries. Nonetheless, bearing these qualifications in mind, it is worth noting that in 1979, Tuvalu life expectancy at birth was lower than that in Western Samoa some fifteen years earlier, and that Tuvalu life expectancies were four to seven years lower than those in Niue and Fiji. Children's mortality rates, particularly for males, were also less favorable than those found in Fiji or Niue.[5] Although the apparent fall in child mortality since 1973 is encouraging, it is sobering to realize that at the time our data on healing practices were gathered, one child out of ten failed to survive to age two in Tuvalu as a whole. Despite local Tuvaluan attempts to maintain their health and to provide a clean living environment, the local health status is clearly more problematic than its surface appearance would indicate.

Economic conditions, diet, and sanitation practices all affect overall health in Tuvalu. Also important are disease and injury patterns, which are related to local life-style both as cause and effect. Our description below of these ethnographic factors is necessarily brief, but more comprehensive information is available in Chambers (1975).

Starvation during extended periods of drought was the most serious threat to community survival in precontact times. The Nanumean community coped by resorting to institutionalized infanticide to limit population size, stockpiling coconuts at the first sign of drought, rationing food on a community basis during the period of scarcity, and, in extreme circumstances, by moving a portion of the population to a remote part of the atoll to use the resources there. Today imported food is of increasing importance and may act as a buffer against shortages of subsistence foods caused by periods of poor fishing conditions, storms, or drought. But shipping services are not always regular or reliable either, and the island store is frequently short of, or out of, major imports such as flour, rice, and sugar. People have substantial sums of money at their disposal since overseas workers (primarily in Banaba and Nauru, and on ships) remit cash home regularly, effectively enlarging the community's resource base. Despite this, locally produced foods which are not within the cash economy—most importantly, fish, coconut, taro, *pulaka,* and breadfruit —remain staples of the daily diet. Sharing and nonmonetary exchange are widespread practices equalizing access to local and imported foods, with the result that all Nanumean households normally have adequate supplies of staple foods. As far as we can determine, neither malnutrition nor overconsumption of refined foods is a current problem on Nanumea.

Awareness of the importance of sanitation is high. Communal latrines built out over the reef on the island's leeward side preserve the water table from contamination and are hygenic in regard to both flies and animals. The lagoon and its sandy foreshore are also used occasionally as latrines, however, most commonly by children. People bathe at least daily in the sea. Slightly saline well water is commonly used for washing clothing and for rinsing after bathing. Drinking water caught from the metal roofs of public buildings is stored in cement cisterns in the village center and dispensed daily. In times of drought when the cisterns run dry, well water (normally considered unpleasantly saline) is substituted for cooking and drinking. This is supplemented by drinking coconuts.

Introduced diseases took their toll in Tuvalu in the nineteenth and early twentieth centuries. Tuberculosis, measles, influenza, whooping cough, and dysentery, as well as yaws and syphilis, were all important contributors to the general decline in health in Tuvalu during this era.[6] Particularly since the Second World War, medical department programs have greatly reduced the impact of these diseases; and of those listed above, only influenza epidemics are currently a health threat on a large scale. Epidemic diseases, of course, remain potential problems. In 1974, during our residence on the island, complications following from a dengue fever outbreak resulted in several deaths.

Infection is a constant possibility for any wound. Small cuts, particularly those from pandanus thorns, usually fester to some extent. Children especially are plagued by small infected sores which develop from cuts, scratches, and insect bites. Ciguatera fish poisoning is also endemic, but not severe compared to its frequency on other Pacific islands. Nanumeans assert that fish poisoning was much more prevalent after the Second World War and in the 1950s than it is at present.[7] Accidental injuries, ranging from falls, cuts, and burns to drowning, occur from time to time and the lack of sophisticated treatment facilities often makes their effects more serious or fatal.

Filariasis was a serious health problem from at least the time of the earliest descriptive reports in the 1870s, and continued to be so until a government-sponsored eradication campaign was effectively mounted against it in the 1970s. The serious effects of this disease in Tuvalu have been discussed by Kennedy (1931, 251) in relation to traditional Vaitupuan concepts of physiology and anatomy. Kennedy believed that the majority of bodily disorders in Tuvalu in about 1930 were "wholly dependent on or aggravated by filariasis." Blood tests made two decades later on Nanumea showed that 50 percent of adult Nanumeans showed either clinical signs of filariasis, or positive blood smears, or both (Venner 1944, 963). Venner also noted, with some surprise, that he found no correlation between the number of microfilaria in the blood smears of individuals and the extent to which they suffered obvious filarial effects such as elephantiasis. Since filariasis apparently has a wide-ranging effect of the lymphatic system, this disease most likely contributes more than just swollen limbs to Tuvaluan health problems.

Although the mortality statistics cited previously indicate that Tuvaluan health has improved in the last decade, disease and injury are nonetheless a constant part of life for Nanumeans and require their active attention for treatment. In an extended survey of Nanumean activity patterns carried out in 1973-74 (reported in detail in Chambers 1975, 175-78), adults reported that a significant portion of their time was lost to illness. Data obtained from the members of nineteen sample households indicated that men aged forty-five and over were particularly likely to be incapacitated by illness or to be occupied in treatment for it. Men of this age in the sample spent, on average, the equivalent of one and a half hours per day in this manner. For women over the age of thirty, the equivalent average was about one hour per day. These relatively high figures for time occupied in illness seem to be due in part to the frequent introduction of colds or mild viral infections which spread rapidly following most visits by ships (ships called at intervals of about three to four weeks during 1973-74).

CAUSES OF ILLNESS AND DEATH

Beliefs about causes of illness and death are crucial in determining the decisions people make about which practitioner to seek help from and which therapy to use. Illness etiologies are also reflected in the repertoire of therapies available in a given society. As Glick (1967, 36, quoted in Foster 1976, 774-75) has noted:

> The most important fact about an illness in most medical systems is not the underlying pathological process but the underlying cause. This is such a central consideration that most diagnoses prove to be statements about causation, and most treatments, responses against particular causal agents.

In Nanumea, the underlying cause of many illnesses involves a realm of nonmaterial superordinate power. While it is not our intention here to discuss Nanumean cosmological beliefs or religious concepts in detail, a brief outline of some of the facets relevant to illness etiologies is useful.

Belief in a superordinate realm of power and spiritual beings is widespread in Nanumea. For most people these beliefs find their common expression in membership and participation in the Tuvalu Church, a protestant church originally founded by the London Missionary Society. Belief in superordinate powers and beings of a distinctly Tuvaluan nature is also important for many people. For some, these powers or beings have been largely amalgamated into a Christian framework; for others, the two realms are kept relatively distinct. The Tuvaluan realm includes, for most Nanumeans, beings *(aitu)* who are sometimes, but not exclusively, conceptualized as spirits of the dead. These beings can be contacted through proper ritual and they assist or harm people in a variety of ways. In the context of illness and healing, *aitu* may play a role either in the etiology of the illness or in healing. Other manifestations of superordinate power include its use in sorcery (the deliberate manipulation of such power by an individual to harm another person), in healing (where diagnostic and therapeutic procedures may draw on it), and in a variety of magical practices designed to secure a goal (e.g. an increased catch of fish) through ritual and verbal manipulation of such power.[8]

A distinction between this supernatural realm and the natural world was drawn by Kennedy[9] in his discussion of illness and healing therapies used in the Tuvalu community of Vaitupu. He asserted (1931, 247):

> It appears that in pre-Christian times, most sickness could be ascribed to causes more or less natural. That is to say, a theory could be advanced by the practitioner *(tufunga [tufuga])* of any particular healing cult to account for the sickness, and on this theory he would base his treatment. If the treatment proved ineffectual, the patient would usually be taken by his family to a practitioner with a totally different theory, and consequently with a different method of treatment. . . . If all such natural methods of treatment failed, it was assumed that the persistent disease was the result of some supernatural agency.

It is not clear from Kennedy's comments whether he felt that Tuvaluan theories of disease causation embodied the distinction he draws between "natural" and "supernatural." He seems to assume a more or less universal dichotomy between natural and supernatural, in line with a western scientific worldview. Yet this distinction does not seem to accord closely with Nanumean (and probably Tuvaluan) theories of the natural order of things as we understand them. Not only is there no term in Nanumean for "supernatural," but there does not appear to be a contrasting concept of "natural." For instance, those illnesses and therapies which draw on or result from the superordinate realm are part of the world as it is conceived by most Nanumeans. The superordinate powers that can be utilized in a malevolent way to harm people can also be used for good, in healing. While there is great variation in the extent to which individuals are interested in this realm of power and feel it is appropriate to use it today, few people (even Christian ministers) deny the existence of this domain. It is "natural" and it is part of the Nanumean construction of reality. This does not imply, however, that Nanumeans make no distinction between the everyday realm and the superordinate realm. In healing practices, for instance, there is a clear diagnostic progression from simple routine causes to more complex ones involving superordinate powers.

Most illnesses *(mahaki)* are assumed to have a physical cause. Minor afflictions like coughs *(tale)*, diarrhoea *(sasana)*, sores *(foge)*,[10] boils *(fakafoa)*, stomachaches *(tinae mamae)*, headaches *(piho mamae)*, sores in the mouth *(gutu)*, colds, and other mild viral infections are understood to happen periodically to almost everyone. If they are troublesome they can be treated with an appropriate therapy from the indigenous or the western medical repertoires, but often they are simply suffered through without treatment. Illnesses considered to be *mahaki* also include those with more serious symptoms, such as fever *(vevela)*, alternate chills and fever *(fiva)*, convulsions *(polepole)*, communicable diseases such as chicken pox/shingles or measles *(misela)*, as well as arthritis *(gugu)*. Fish poisoning (ciguatera) is also attributed to a purely physical cause. *Mahaki* illness is treated with utmost pragmatism: the illness is either to be endured or its symptoms ameliorated by the application of appropriate therapy. Once the illness has been diagnosed as a normal physical one, its possible physiological cause is of little concern to Nanumeans. What does continue to interest them is the choice of therapy and its application.

Illnesses with a component we might deem "magical" or which involve the realm of superordinate power can manifest the same physical symptoms as those that appear to have a simple physical cause, so that Nanumeans usually do not find it possible to distinguish clearly between them at the outset of a problem. Suspicions of sorcery are characteristically aroused when a complaint lasts an unusually long time or when conventional therapies do not seem to help. The existence of sorcery-induced illness, *mahaki māhei,* can only be confirmed and treated by a local medical practitioner *(tino fai vailākau).*[11] Although local practitioners usually provide some information about who is believed responsible for the sorcery and why it has been employed, identification of the source of sorcery is not their main concern, nor is it that of the sick person. Nor does this knowledge determine the therapy employed. Furthermore, knowing these aspects of the "cause" of sorcery is not sufficient to "cure" the problem. The effectiveness of therapy for a sorcery-induced illness rests in the relative strength of the spiritual power that the practitioner can invoke. Because sorcery often aims at the death of the victim, the diagnosis of an illness as being sorcery-induced means that it is regarded as potentially more serious than the symptoms themselves might otherwise seem to warrant. As will be described below, sorcery can cause illness or death for the individual at whom it is specifically aimed, as well as to people in close association with that person. If a spell is lodged in a particular place like a house, anyone regularly in the vicinity can be affected.

Magic can also cause physical and mental disability or death in another manner. Magic to increase productivity in fishing or other economic pursuits is bound tightly by rules and regulations. The exact nature of these varies between individual practitioners but commonly involves prohibitions. The rules may restrict individual action, as in prohibitions against urinating or eating at sea, or they may affect the treatment of some tool or piece of equipment, as in a prohibition against letting a fishing net, on which a spell has been cast, touch the ground. Nanumeans say that those who employ magic are dealing with power so strong that inept or careless use of it can be fatal to themselves or their children. It was routinely pointed out to us that the men who were renowned for their use of magic in fishing inevitably had managed to produce no children of their own, or had lost their children through illness or accidental injury. The use of magic can also place an individual in situations that might be beyond his or her ability to cope with. For example, nets or outrigger canoes that have had a spell placed on them are said to sometimes attract huge fish, much larger than intended, which may ram the canoe and kill the fisherman or otherwise injure him.

Some magic spells are said to involve a pact with a particular *aitu* 'spirit'. These spirits are known to be capricious and quick to anger. To break a rule *(soli te fakatonuga)* insisted on by the spirit, whether purposely or inadvertently, can anger the spirit and induce it to mete out a harsh punishment. Nanumeans also characterize *aitu* as easily fed up or irritated *(fiu)* by the constant requests made of them by people who practice magic *(fai vai* or *fai aitu)*. Angry *aitu* are dangerous, and frequently cause an accident involving the practitioner of magic.

During our period of field research, the deaths of two men were widely attributed to their misuse of magical power. V, a middle-aged man in apparent good health, was found unconscious and badly injured at the base of the coconut tree which he climbed daily to collect coconut sap or "toddy." He had apparently fallen while climbing. He died several days later without regaining consciousness. His death was attributed to cerebral hemorrhage by the western-trained doctor resident on the island. Village rumors, however, linked the death to the anger of the spirit who had assisted V with his toddy magic. V was believed by some to be able to boil fresh toddy into toddy molasses with no significant reduction in the volume in the amount of fresh toddy begun with. People remembered how he had always insisted on boiling the toddy down himself, rather than letting his wife or daughters do this work as was customary. They speculated that one day he had been careless and allowed the toddy to boil over, thus angering the spirit which had been helping him. When he later fell from his toddy tree, some people were sure the spirit had pushed him to his death.

In the second case, death came through illness. M, a seemingly healthy man in his early fifties, developed a flu-like sickness. After a few days, he suffered convulsions that culminated in a stroke which paralyzed the right side of his body. In the interval before M's death, a kinsman borrowed his canoe for fishing and was surprised to see four fish swimming toward the canoe in a "crazy" manner. The man interpreted this to mean that M had put a magic spell on the canoe (*hae vaka,* lit. "tie [knots in the] canoe"). On returning to shore he warned the sick man's family to cut all the lashings on the outrigger canoe so that the magic spell could be broken. The sick man's family refused, saying that M did not practice fishing magic. Within a few days, to his family's sorrow and the local western-trained doctor's surprise, M was dead. Widespread local opinion was that he had been injured by his fishing magic *(pakia i tana hae vaka).*

There do not seem to be any fixed characteristics that automatically indicate that a death is due to the misuse of magic, or to sorcery. In fact, even when this interpretation is widely rumored in the community the deceased's kin, as well as the community's Christian leaders, usually maintain otherwise. The deaths of elderly people and children are not usually attributed to supernatural causes except when those individuals are closely related to a "known" magical practitioner. Though the deaths of men who are middle-aged and ostensibly healthy (and for whom death is thus unexpected) do tend to be related to contact with the superordinate realm, they are not always given this explanation. In the following case death was assigned a purely routine cause, in spite of the rather unusual circumstances surrounding the death, and the numerous explanatory dreams connected with it.

The body of P, a middle-aged man known for his fishing knowledge, was found floating in the ocean near the village. Mouth-to-mouth resuscitation failed to revive him and the western-trained doctor pronounced him dead, ostensibly from drowning. The community was shocked by this sudden accident but people remembered that a traditional practitioner once told P that he would die at sea with none of his children present. A local healer also recounted a dream he had had the previous night. He had seen a woman carrying P's body. Now, he said, the meaning of this dream was clear; it foretold P's death. As far as we were able to ascertain, neither sorcery nor fishing magic nor a spirit's power was believed to be implicated in P's accident. His death did not go unexplained, however. A week after he was buried, P's spirit appeared to a neighbor and described the circumstances of his death. He had gone to bathe in the sea and while bathing had suffered a bad pain in his right shoulder. This had caused that arm to stiffen at his side and had affected his balance. He struggled to reach shore but fell and then drowned.

Love magic can also produce striking physical symptoms in its victims, in addition to the intended psychological changes. E, an unmarried young woman in her late teens, fainted in church one Sunday. By evening her parents, worried that her breathing was abnormal, sent for the doctor. Her breathing and pulse seemed all right to him, but the doctor agreed that she seemed strangely quiet and withdrawn. E complained that her abdomen hurt, but the doctor's inspection revealed nothing and he recommended she have a good night's sleep. Her withdrawn behavior continued the next day, but by the following morning the cause of her problem had become clear to her family; she told her father she could think of nothing else than a particular young man, and that she was longing to see his face. Obvious physical effects, though certainly not uncommon, do not always result from love magic incidents. Sometimes nothing but an uncharacteristic change in behavior or mental attitude shows that love magic has been done.

Nanumeans also believe that a spirit, if sufficiently provoked, can strike an individual dead. Sweeping with a broom after dark, calling out loudly in the bush, and chasing dogs with a stick at night were actions mentioned as capable of enraging the spirits. As evidence for the need to be careful not to offend an *aitu,* the case of L was described to us. This woman had been found one morning lying on the ground, dead, with a stick clutched in one hand. She was believed to have been using the stick to chase dogs away from her bitch in heat during the night. She should have thrown stones instead, people said, so as not to anger the spirits.

Becoming startled *(fakapoi)* or taken by surprise can also cause the onset of serious health problems. T, a woman in her late fifties, was working in the bush in the late afternoon when she was suddenly startled by a woman calling to her that it was time to go home. By the time she reached home she had developed a bad headache *(mahoko te piho),* and the next day her face was twisted, her mouth pulled to one side *(peke te gutu).* The western-trained doctor diagnosed her problem as a pinched nerve. T remained in Nanumea's hospital for about a month but the doctor's injections did little for her. In fact, her condition continued to worsen. She was unable to sleep, she talked incessantly, she cried, she gobbled down her food. She talked a lot about dying. Eventually she was widely regarded as being possessed by a spirit *(fakahegihegi).* The pastor prayed with her in the hope of freeing her from the devil *(tiapolo)* that he himself believed responsible for the possession. People began to gossip about her stated desire to eat people and drew half-hearted connections, which never amounted to anything, between her words and the sudden death of an old man, and another death by drowning.

The stereotypical symptoms of spirit possession *(fakahegihegi* or, more generally, *fakavalevale)*[12] are rather different from those which T exhibited, however. They include (1) wandering around aimlessly, not knowing where one is going, not following the accustomed paths; (2) talking a strange language, often said to be part-Samoan; and (3) seeing people who are dead, believing they are real and trying to accompany them to an often dangerous place, such as to the top of a tree or on a nonexistent canoe across the lagoon.

The pastor usually provides effective help in these cases. His mere presence may itself produce a cure, or he may intervene, often by changing the possessed person's name. This common practice is believed to alter, in some manner, the link between the affected person and the superordinate realm and to result in amelioration of the condition. Alternatively, therapy may be sought from a traditional practitioner. Interestingly, *aitu* possess women but usually entice or seduce men.

Strict Christian and lay explanations for mental disturbance in Nanumea are somewhat at odds, but for many people they seem to coexist in an unsystematic manner. *Aitu* are believed capable of causing people to do dangerous and crazy things, such as walking straight into the sea until the waters close overhead. This was the fate of one man in the 1960s, and it was widely believed that he had had extensive dealings with *aitu* and that they had deranged him. The church condemns all dealings with *aitu* and one explanation of this man's death made this connection clear; he had walked into the sea because "his cup was too full of sin, he was possessed" *(ko tō pī te ipu i agahala, fakahegihegi)*. Thus, from the Nanumean Christian point of view, such injuries and the mental disturbances felt to underlie them are a punishment meted out by God for practicing magic rather than the result of insufficient control over the power involved. The full moon is also believed to aggravate the symptoms of the mentally ill, however, and one traditional practitioner sometimes uses the moon in his treatment of mental disorders.

Finally, Nanumeans recognize that some disabilities seem to affect several members of a family. During the Second World War military doctors stationed on Nanumea investigated the incidence of filariasis in the local population and the characteristics of its mosquito vector. They found that Nanumeans believed the swollen limbs caused by filariasis were a "disease that runs in certain families," and had nothing to do with mosquitoes (Venner 1944, 955–56). We found, however, that this notion of family susceptibility was not used to explain several cases of clubfoot *(vaepeke)* which affected some males in one extended family. Instead, each instance was explained separately as retributive punishment. In one case, the child's mother, while pregnant, reportedly teased a boy about his father's clubfoot and was punished by having her own son born with one. In another case, a man ordered his pregnant daughter-in-law's younger brother to leave his house, ostensibly because the boy's handicap might also come to affect the unborn child. The infant was in fact born with a clubfoot, but this was seen to be retribution for the man's unkindness rather than a family affliction.

With this overlapping set of rationales, coming to understand the cause of an illness, physical or mental disability, or death can require time. An essential part of the process is the application of an initial diagnostic label, the use of a likely therapy, and the subsequent evaluation of its effects. If the diagnosis changes, other alternative therapies may then be applied in sequence. Though therapeutic practices are part of the cure, they also play an important role in diagnosing the causes of illness.

USE OF WESTERN MEDICAL SERVICES AND THERAPIES

Western medical services of varying degrees of sophistication and comprehensiveness have been available to Nanumeans since the early days of this century. In 1909 the assistant high commissioner, Western Pacific High Commission, alarmed to discover that deaths outnumbered births on some of the Ellice Islands, requested that an expatriate doctor be assigned to the group. In his correspondence with the high commissioner he continued to lobby for this service, and he also persuaded the island communities to contribute toward the cost of the doctor's support. In 1910 the first resident doctor arrived. He was based in Funafuti, the administrative center of the Ellice Islands, where he ran a small hospital and periodically toured the outer islands (Western Pacific High Commission 1909). Judging from official correspondence, the early doctors' most important task in local opinion was surgery: people suffering from filariasis and glandular tuberculosis made their own way to Funafuti seeking operations to remove the swollen areas. Surgery (*tipi,* lit. "cut, make incision") had been part of the medical repertoire in the Ellice Islands for some time, however. Though western surgical techniques may inherently have had some advantages over their traditional counterparts, the enthusiastic use of the doctors' services did not result simply from a local appreciation of these advantages. Following the establishment of a British protectorate in 1892, a general ban had been placed on the practice of all "native medicine," including surgery and abortion (Kennedy 1931, 238, 264). This prohibition, although it was never rigidly enforced, created a situation in which western medicine ostensibly could flourish without overt competition.

As successive doctors implemented programs to eradicate or contain such scourges as tuberculosis, yaws, syphilis, and filariasis, local belief in the utility of western medicine was largely validated. By 1916 there was a hospital on Nanumea itself and a system of direct, though rudimentary, medical care was soon instituted, with locally resident dressers being given basic western medical training and supplies. Infrequent and slow transport limited both the doctors' supervision of outer island staff and their ability to assist with difficult cases. During these early years, the most effective aspect of western medicine was the development of broad programs aimed at particular diseases rather than the treatment of individual cases.

From these beginnings, western medical services have expanded considerably. Early in this century local dressers did little more than supply antiseptic and sticking plasters. In recent decades Tuvalu men have been trained as doctors at the Fiji Medical School, and both dressers and trained nurses now serve the outer island communities. Medical programs against yaws and syphilis have long been successful, and more recently, efforts to combat tuberculosis and eliminate filariasis have been effective. In the late 1960s a family planning program was implemented and local women were trained in maternal and child health care. Under the supervision of the island nurse, these women run the prenatal and postnatal clinics where babies' growth is charted, mothers' health monitored, and supplementary vitamins, powdered milk, and birth control apparatus are dispensed. Before 1976, the district hospital in Funafuti and the larger colony hospital in Tarawa, in the Gilbert Islands, served as backups for the local hospitals in each community. At present, the main hospital in Funafuti fills this role. The local hospitals remain the focal point of western medical services in each community, however.

The Nanumean hospital compound, built in the late sixties, is located a short distance from the main village on leased land. In addition to a substantial house which serves as the doctor's residence, the hospital compound contains a number of houses for staff and patients, a maternity clinic, and a dispensary. Outpatients are treated daily in the dispensary and, although medicines may occasionally come into short supply due to shipping difficulties, patients usually have the benefit of a sophisticated array of western medications. Seriously ill patients—those requiring isolation from the community or the doctor's close supervision—move into residence at the hospital, accompanied by as many family members as are needed to provide for their physical and emotional needs. Most babies, and virtually all first babies, are born in the hospital's maternity clinic under the supervision of the nurse.

Medical department reports (Gilbert and Ellice Islands Colony 1944–67) document the increasing use Nanumeans have made of the western medical services available to them on the island. Between 1950 and 1968, the number of inpatients treated held roughly steady, ranging between ninety-two and twenty-five annually. Outpatient numbers averaged about two thousand per year in the 1950s, about five thousand per year in the 1960s, and rose to a high of twelve thousand annually in 1966 and 1967. In December 1973 our brief survey of outpatient treatment found an average of nineteen outpatients seen per day at the dispensary. If this figure is representative, and it is probably only a rough guide, an annual outpatient figure of at least six thousand (about six visits per capita) would be indicated for 1973. Home visits made by the medical personnel and attendance at the family planning and maternal and child health clinics would boost this figure further. Dispensary records show that simple medicines are most commonly given to outpatients.[13] Gentian violet swabs are the usual treatment for all types of skin infections, lacerations, and abrasions, while aspirin is dispensed for body aches and cough syrup for bronchial complaints. Penicillin, zinc oxide, and sulphadimidine tablets are also dispensed, however, and patients with chronic diseases receive a variety of specific medications.

Many Nanumeans use the western medical services as their first line of therapy, attending the dispensary to obtain treatment for sores, cuts, and pain relief. In our survey, reported in Table 1, small sores are the most common complaint brought to the dispensary for treatment, followed by wounds of various types and severity. These ailments, together with the treatment of chronic diseases, accounted for about 60 percent of the outpatient cases during the four days of the survey.

In cases of serious illness, western-trained medical staff are always summoned as far as we are aware. Local therapies are most often used to treat minor complaints or those for which western medicine had previously been used but was believed to have been ineffectual. Thus a cut, headache, or child's fever often might be treated first with a local remedy, but if the symptoms persist or worsen western medical care is usually sought. Similarly, if the western-trained doctor's medicine is judged not to work or if he has been unable to pinpoint the problem, help is sought from a traditional healer. The Nanumean approach to healing is essentially pragmatic and people often use several therapies in combination.

The case of T illustrates some characteristic attitudes to treating injuries and to choosing (and mixing) therapies. A misplaced hammer blow had smashed open the upper side of T's thumb. The wound was given no special care and after two days had become badly infected. Her thumb as well as the thumb side of her hand was swollen to twice its normal size and was red and very painful. T sought treatment at the hospital but the medicine put on the wound stung so badly that she washed it off on her return home and applied coconut oil instead. She had been instructed to

Table 1. Outpatient Dispensary Treatment, Nanumea, 17–20 December 1973

Type of Problem		Cases
Wounds	Lacerated wound	10
	Bite	1
	Abrasion	2
	Burn	2
Sores	Small sores	20
	Abscess	1
	Boil	2
Respiratory Infections	Cough	6
	Bronchitis/Pneumonia	2
	Common cold	2
Pain	Joint pain	3
	Abdominal pain	2
	Urinary tract infection	1
	Sore arm	1
	Gastric pain (liver)	1
Miscellaneous	Diarrhoea	1
	Fish poisoning	2
	Fever	1
	Enlarged lymph node/groin	1
	Typhoid immunization	1
	Chronic diseases (6 indiv.)	14

Total: 76 cases treated. Source: field research

return to the hospital in three days and, since her thumb was, if anything, more infected by then, she did so. She received an injection of penicillin, her hand was bandaged and she was told to return again in four days, on Monday morning. When we saw T during the weekend, she complained that her thumb was still painfully infected and was interfering with her work. Her hand was now so swollen that the wound itself looked as though a hunk had been bitten out of it.

Since she was unwilling to return to the dispensary earlier than she had been instructed to, but was worried about her hand, we gave her some antibiotic salve and bandage to use. When we saw her later that same day, she had washed the wound and applied a poultice of chopped hibiscus leaves to it, covered over with a whole leaf. Two of her close relatives had recommended this as a sure cure and, responding as we had to her worry, urged her to try it. The following day, Monday, T anointed her hand with our antibiotic salve and covered it over with a fresh leaf poultice. The thumb had begun to itch and she could tell that it was getting better. She did not return to the dispensary, though she would have done so if there had been no sign of improvement. Eventually her thumb healed well without complications.

Nanumeans seem to have only a vague understanding of the role germs play in infection and the reasons hygiene is so important. The care usually taken to prevent infection and its spread is minimal. Like most people the world over, Nanumeans are oriented mainly to obtaining effective care for their health problems as they occur. Because western medicines tend to be effective in relieving symptoms with a simple physical cause, they are widely used and appreciated. But, because even the simplest medications are only obtainable from the medical staff and therapy has to be sought at a given time, largely in a particular place, and usually from nonrelatives (that is, from the nurse/dresser/doctor at the hospital or clinic), western medical therapies are not always the first ones used, especially for minor ailments. In the treatment of sorcery-induced illnesses, or those that stem from other applications of superordinate power, western medicines and therapies are regarded as ineffective.

TRADITIONAL MEDICAL PRACTICES

Today Nanumeans use a wide repertoire of nonwestern healing practices to which we have here applied the general label "traditional." Many of these therapies actually do seem to stem from the intertwined corpus of religious beliefs, magical techniques, and medical knowledge that predated intensive western contact. The therapeutic rituals used to treat sorcery-induced illness seem particularly traditional in this strict sense because of their close fit with what is known of precontact religious practices. It is more difficult to determine the extent to which such physiological remedies as massage *(popō)*, pressure application *(kukumi)*, heat application *(tutu)*, bloodletting *(kikini)*, surgery *(tipi)*, and herbal medicines *(vailākau* or *vai)* embody precontact practices, since they have also figured in the practice of western medicine. However, the specialized surgical tools and techniques documented by Kennedy (1931, 236–46) half a century ago on Vaitupu strongly suggest that both surgery and bloodletting were indigenous medical practices. This conclusion is supported by Nanumean accounts of ancestors who variously survived or succumbed to surgery or its complications, dating via genealogy to about 1870. The large number of named techniques for massage and pressure application recorded by Kennedy (1931, 250–55) indicate that the existence of these therapies also probably antedates the introduction of western medicine to Tuvalu.

By contrast, purely herbal medicines may be a more recent borrowing. Kennedy (1931, 248) reported that "medicine potions, herbal or otherwise, were never prescribed" traditionally on Vaitupu and that herbal cures in use at the time of his research (the mid-1920s) had been introduced from Fiji. The main practitioners of traditional therapies in Nanumea in 1973–74 similarly did not use herbal remedies, though these were widely known in the community and one other person made something of a specialty of using them. The preeminent traditional medical practitioner *(tino fai vai)* on the atoll conceptualizes medicines as coming from two contrasting sources: *lau* 'leaves' and *hua* 'liquid or juice made by squeezing things'. Leaves are a key ingredient in all Nanumean therapies against illness caused by superordinate power, and are used for treating some illnesses with simple physical causes as well. As far as we are aware, however, *hua* is not used in therapy involving superordinate power.

In precontact times, ancestral spirits *(feao* or *atuāfale)* were propitiated by the senior male of each extended family group and provided assistance to their own descendants. These spirits could be asked for information about the cause of an illness as well as about future or distant happenings. They also could confer protection *(puipui)* during a trip, cause illness in others, or work love magic on them. The victim of an ancestral spirit's power would consult his or her own spirit, requesting therapeutic help and protection. The two *feao* would be drawn into combat and the victor would be the one with the greater spirit power. The spirit communicated with the buzzing sounds made by a cricket *(ligoligo)*. Though anyone could hear it, only the senior family member who propitiated the spirit could understand the meaning of its sound. Every family group thus had its own source of superordinate power and its own "medicine" *(vailākau)* which could be used either defensively or aggressively to the advantage of its members. Unlike the rights to chieftainship and other political roles, as well as skills like outrigger canoe building, this therapeutic system was not parcelled out as a specialty to any particular lineage. Extended family groups also appear to have been relatively self-sufficient in the practice of massage *(popō)*, pressure application *(kukumi)*, and midwifery *(fakafānau)*, including the massage skills *(popō tinae)* used in pregnancy. It seems likely to us, however, that the knowledge involved in these therapies was generally shared and standardized throughout the community in spite of its intrafamily practice.

According to Kennedy (1931, 247), two sorts of medical specialists practiced in precontact Vaitupu. *Vaka atua,* literally "canoe/vessel [of the] gods," were able to cure illness by virtue of their rapport with a particular island deity. *Tufuga* 'skilled practitioners' specialized in the treatment of disease through surgery, heat application, bloodletting, and massage. Today in Nanumea *vaka atua* is an archaic term, and while the word *tufuga* for expert or specialist is known, it seems seldom to be used to denote a traditional medical practitioner. One hears instead the designation *tino fai vai* (or *tagata fai vai*). *Tino fai vai* today use therapies designed for simple physical complaints as well as more complex procedures to assist with illnesses linked to superordinate power.

Nanumeans say there are several different traditions of indigenous medicine *(matāvai)*. All of the important traditional practitioners on Nanumea in 1973–74 claimed to trace their knowledge originally to a Fijian from "Malekula" village, who passed his knowledge and power to an indigenous practitioner at Vaitupu early in this century. The Vaitupuan practitioner then transmitted in his turn two systems of *vailākau* 'medicine', one to his daughter and another to his sons. Through marital connections several descendants of the Vaitupu practitioner now live and practice in Nanumea. Practitioners from other traditions also reside on Nanumea, though they were not practicing at the time of our research. These traditions include a medical one derived from the island of Niutao and two other Nanumean varieties. Within these local medical traditions there are both male and female practitioners, though male practitioners are more numerous.

In choosing a local practitioner, people prefer to deal with a relative, however distant, if this is possible. Even when referred to a nonrelative by a nonpracticing kinsman, they appear somewhat hesitant to trust his or her skills. All the well-known practitioners of traditional medicine assert that they use their skills only to benefit people, never to harm them. Nonetheless, they recognize that the power involved in their therapies also could be tapped for malevolent purposes. *"Te vai e lelei, ka ko tino e māhei,"* they say. "The medicine is good, but people are bad."[14] The individuals of whom we heard sorcery allegations did not practice as healers. Interestingly, their own kin maintained these persons' innocence of sorcery on the grounds that they had never been seen to practice magic or to have any of the proper implements about.

We now briefly describe six types of therapy used in Nanumea and the contexts in which they are applied. From this description we will subsequently draw some generalizations about the Nanumean approach to sickness and healing.

Herbal Therapies

A variety of herbal therapies, including both medicinal drinks and externally applied medicines, are known and used today in Nanumea. Characteristically, a specific remedy is concocted to ease a particular condition. The following examples show the range and style of the therapies used:

1. For headache: cut up the stem and leaves of *aluna (Laportea ruderalis)* and put them in water. Dip a cloth in the water and place on the forehead.

2. To hasten recovery from measles by bringing the bumps out faster: have the child chew on the end of an aerial root of pandanus.
3. To counteract the lethal stonefish sting: chop up four *talotalo* (*Crinum asiaticum* L.) leaf shoots and tie them up in a piece of the fibrous matting that protects the young furled coconut leaf. Put this bundle in a small amount of coconut oil and boil it. Make an incision in the foot to the point where the stonefish sting has penetrated and then press the cooled, oily packet onto this cut. The remaining oil is then basted on periodically.

In general, external therapies seem to be more common than internal ones.

Plant materials also provide the ingredients for treating a common childhood illness, *kili,* in which the afflicted child is feverish, writhing with pain, crying, and cannot be comforted. In treating *kili,* an herbal mixture serves both as a diagnostic and a therapeutic agent. In the case we observed, the child's mother was given a breadfruit leaf containing a mixture of chopped leaves and coconut oil and was instructed to rub this mixture all over the child's body, cover the child with a cloth, and leave it wrapped for several hours. The child was to continue to sleep on these cloths for several days and not to bathe in the meantime. This therapy is believed to work by drawing out the fever *(vela)* from the child's body, as evidenced by the red and black blotches, resembling leaf stains, that appeared in several hours and signaled the end of the illness.

Plant-based concoctions are also used to produce an abortion by combining ingestion of the concoction with abdominal beating, pressure and/or the application of bottles of hot water to the woman's back.

In some herbal therapies, ritualized elements are important. Thus, one therapy for cuts and scratches prescribes that two seedheads of the grass *mouku tū* (*Eleusine india* L.) be put together so that the four parts point out to the "four corners of the earth." They are then dipped in oil which is applied to the injury. A similar preoccupation with ritual is seen in a cure for diarrhoea where the sick person must himself watch the herb preparation being made.

Heat Application (Tutu)

Kennedy (1931, 248–50) described heat application (which he called cautery) as a common therapy for disorders ranging from filarial swelling to digestive upsets, abdominal pains, bruises, and aching teeth. The treatment consists of touching the end of a glowing roll of cloth or bark briefly, usually repeatedly, to the surface of the skin. Kennedy found that on Vaitupu the hot punk usually was applied to several selected points above or below the actual affected area, though it was applied directly to treat bruises, toothache, and swollen scrotum. We observed heat application in Nanumea on only one occasion.

Massage (Popō) *and Pressure Application* (Kukumi)

Massage is perhaps the most commonly used therapy on Nanumea, one that is applied routinely to the common injuries and sprains incurred in daily life, as well as to a variety of specific health problems. It is used by the main traditional practitioners, by midwives, by therapists who specialize in massage, as well as by ordinary people. Kennedy (1931, 252–54) lists fifteen types of massage (termed *puke* in Vaitupu), all of which he says were restricted in use to people skilled in massage. Both in Vaitupu and in contemporary Nanumea massage aims at softening stiff, hardened (and thus painful) areas.

The nonspecialist use of massage and pressure application usually seeks to relieve transitory pain by direct attention to the affected area. In one case we observed, a child returned from school with a mildly sprained hand. Her mother massaged her hand for about fifteen minutes, applying coconut oil as she rubbed. She then continued to hold the child's hand, exerting moderate pressure, for another ten minutes until the child indicated she had had enough treatment. Massage of a hand, arm, or leg is also a common way of comforting someone who is generally not feeling well. Very gentle massage is also applied intensively to a clubfoot for the first few days after birth in order to straighten it.

A number of Nanumeans are recognized locally for their expertise in using massage as treatment for an ailment in a particular part of the body. They usually are asked to assist relatives with minor and short-term aches and pains. Midwives also administer a specific form of abdominal massage *(popō tinae)* during the last months of pregnancy as part of their routine prenatal care. While the mother-to-be lies on her back on the floor, the midwife spreads her hands on each side of the woman's abdomen near the hip. Pressing inward, with a jiggling motion, she works her hands upwards until the abdomen falls through them. This is repeated, beginning at different points, for about ten minutes. Its goal is to further an easy birth by making sure that the baby is lying straight in the womb. The benefits of this treatment are certainly psychological as well as physical. While she massages, the midwife also discusses with the woman any problems or worries the latter might have, and describes to her the baby's development and progress toward birth.

In the hands of a specialist, massage becomes a more complicated therapy. He or she must determine whether the sick person's pain is the result of sorcery *(vailākau māhei)* or is simply a physical sickness *(mahaki)* because each requires a different sort of massage. Thus the specialist first palpates the sore area. If he can feel a hardness or swelling (termed a *malaga)*, he simply massages on that spot to soften it. Sorcery-induced ailments involve an invisible power (not an object) residing in the body. These can hide *(fakalilolilo)* from the practitioner by being located elsewhere than the apparent site of pain. Thus the actual place where the magic power resides *(momea e noho i ai)* must be found and then pressure *(kukumi)* or hard massage *(popō)* applied to keep it stationary. Once the power is prevented from jumping around, the person's pain stops and, in the simplest cases, the power departs.

The shoulder and thigh muscles are believed to be likely places for sorcery power to hide. In one case we observed, the young daughter of a woman undergoing treatment for sorcery suddenly began to cry from a stomachache. The traditional practitioner's assistant first massaged her stomach with the specially prepared coconut oil (a spell had been placed on it) that was readily to hand, and then the practitioner felt the stomach. Abruptly, he instructed his assistant to squeeze the girl's knee while he continued to feel her stomach. In a moment he reported that the stomach muscles had softened, indicating the therapy had worked. Though the stomachache ostensibly had been caused by sorcery, this instant cure was possible because the sorcery was directed to the child's mother rather than to the child herself. More complex healing practices, which are described below, provide the only appropriate treatment for a person such as the mother in this case.

Bloodletting (Kikini)

Kikini (lit. "beat") is a form of surface bloodletting accomplished by lightly striking the affected part with a shark tooth–tipped instrument. Kennedy mentions it as one of several surgical techniques in Vaitupu, one that was believed to be useful for treating bruises, headache, gumboil, itch, and early-stage filarial swelling. In Nanumea, we observed a *kikini* treatment for *gugu* (arthritis, rheumatism, synovitis) on the swollen index finger joint of a man's hand. The treatment was performed by one of the community's main traditional practitioners and was repeated about every other day for over a week. A shark tooth–tipped instrument was tapped gently with a wooden mallet ten to fifteen times so as to make many small punctures on the puffy, swollen knuckle area. The blood that appeared was wiped away and the knuckle was carefully examined. The treatment was repeated twice more and then the practitioner carefully anointed *(teitei)* the affected area with specially prepared coconut oil.

Bloodletting was chosen as treatment, we were told, because there was "something bad" *(mea māhei)* in the blood of the swollen area. The *mea māhei* was not considered, in this case, to result from sorcery or other superordinate power. Getting rid of the affected blood allowed the knuckle to recover. Kennedy (1931, 245–46) apparently found this type of bloodletting practiced in essentially the same manner in Vaitupu half a century ago, but his brief account does not describe the physiological rationale behind the treatment. Interestingly, heat application and massage, rather than bloodletting, were the recommended therapies for *gugu* on Vaitupu at that time.

Power Therapies (Vailākau)

Power therapies are required to treat and, to a lesser extent, explain the illnesses caused by sorcery. These illnesses, which are believed to result from malevolent use of superordinate power, can be brought about in two ways. In one, the power is directed at the person. In the other, a specially prepared bottle of coconut oil is buried near one of the posts in the person's house with the goal of afflicting the residents indiscriminately. Though the belief in sorcery-caused illnesses is widespread in Nanumea, and along with it the view that some people in the community use sorcery, no one admits to using magic to cause misfortune to others. As there is no information available from practitioners on the spells and procedures used, our understanding of sorcery is based on observation of the therapies used to "open" *(tatala)* or remove a sorcery spell, and on explanations by healers of their therapies and the characteristic diagnostic signs which lead them to conclude sorcery is involved in a given case. Though we describe below the consistent structure of the therapeutic rituals that are used to treat sorcery, it must be remembered that particular details vary between different practitioners.

Initial diagnosis of sorcery is usually based on information which practitioners say is conveyed to them personally. It may be brought on a visit by a spirit in the night. "The old man (the spirit of her dead father) came to me last night," explained one healer. Other practitioners say they are "informed" *(ni fakailoa mai)* or "see" who is responsible for the sorcery. These phrasings are deliberate, and are not veiled ways of referring to dreams, for dreams *(moemiti)* figure in other ways in conveying information to the specialist. Sometimes a spontaneous dream causes an affected person to seek help from a traditional practitioner. In other cases the practitioner warns the affected person to expect an illuminating dream, which the practitioner then interprets. These dreams usually pinpoint the sorcerer fairly explicitly but they seldom disclose the reasons why the supposed sorcerer should wish to harm the individual. The practitioner himself may also dream about the case. Sometimes he dreams of the person who will soon be seeking help from him and of the details of his case. Other times, a familiar spirit may come to advise about the plants to use in the curing rituals or offer advice or warning.

Although understanding who is responsible seems to be emphasized in the diagnostic stage of superordinate power therapy, this information does not usually provoke a confrontation between the two parties. No pressure is normally put on the suspected sorcerer (if, indeed, he or she is resident on the island at the time) to remove his spell or to cease and desist. There also seems to be little concern to avoid interpersonal disputes so as to prevent sorcery or sorcery allegations. Instead, the traditional practitioner attempts to overcome malevolent magic by the application of a stronger power and makes no attempt to reconcile the parties or mediate their disagreements.

Suspicions of sorcery are treated seriously, however. Since sorcery is forbidden by law as well as condemned by the church, a public accusation of sorcery leads to a court case in which the accused angrily claims he or she has been slandered. Allegations of sorcery are thus very rarely made public. Often the person deemed responsible does not live on the island. When the suspected sorcerer is a local resident, it is more likely that the problem will eventually be aired publicly and find its way to court. The usual pattern is for the person accused of sorcery to use the court case to clear his or her name rather than for the sufferer to prosecute. In any case, all are aware that it is virtually impossible to prove to the satisfaction of the court that sorcery has been done. In one unusual court case, a traditional practitioner who claimed to be able to see in a fire the face of the sorcerer who was alleged to have caused a man's death was told to produce the proof in court. He kindled his fire and again claimed to see the sorcerer's face but the skeptical local court could see nothing and found the accused man innocent, and the practitioner guilty of slander. At the accused sorcerer's request, the practitioner was reprimanded rather than being given a heavy fine.

The therapeutic rituals themselves constitute a three- or four-part series which is performed over the course of a week, or if unsuccessful, over a longer period of time. These are always preceded by a period of diagnosis, often lasting several days, during which the sick person is repeatedly anointed with special coconut oil one or more times a day. The oil contains an infusion of plant materials and, sometimes, grubs. In order that the oil have the requisite potency to be effective the practitioner must be guided by familiar spirits to the correct plants. The oil may also have incantations said over it *(lalau)*.

In cases where a spell is believed to have been put on the house of the sick person, a ritual to counter this spell, termed *te tatalaga o te fale* 'the opening of the house', is performed first. This dramatic ceremony aims at locating and nullifying the malevolent power of a hidden bottle of oil.[15] Several axe heads[16] are heated in a fire until red hot. Then each is brought in turn to a house post, where the practitioner spits coconut oil onto it. If that post is free from the "evil thing" *(mea māhei)*, the oil bursts into flame when it hits the glowing axe. If there is something "wrong" (*fakalavelave,* lit. "problem, trouble"), then there is only smoke. As each post is tested, the used axe head is put into a pot filled with chopped leaves and when all have been used, smoke from this pot is wafted around the house. The sick person and the older members of the household are decorated with protective flower and leaf wreaths. The healer and his assistant are then served a meal and he discusses his findings with the people present. This procedure both illuminates the source of the illness, "the thing injuring him" *(te mea e pakia ai),* and "opens," or renders harmless, the spell, causing the "evil thing" to go elsewhere *(ke olo ki ātea mea māhei).*

The next ritual, termed *te fakapūlou* 'the covering', is aimed at "opening" the power focused specifically on the sick person. One practitioner told us this ritual functions like an X-ray *(fakaata* 'make image', hence 'photograph, X-ray') to determine in which part of the body the evil power lurks. Again, red hot axe heads are used. This time they are circled in turn around the person's head and then near different parts of his body. They flare up as the practitioner spits out oil. A black mark, seen in the flame by the healer, signifies the illness. As they are used the axes are put into a pot full of leaves, and finally coconut oil is poured on top to produce dense, aromatic smoke. The sick person sits near the pot and is covered completely with mats so that the smoke, which is believed to be able to carry the evil power away with it, will be trapped around him. After several minutes the mats are opened, the smoke disperses, and the person is anointed with the healer's coconut oil. Wreaths are then put on the main participants, with the purpose of protecting them against any further possibility of harm. The practitioner and his assistant are given a meal and a gift, perhaps a shirt or towel. Again, there is discussion of what the healer has seen and its meaning, and the patient is given specific instructions for bathing and anointing during the next few days.

If the sorcery has not been fully counteracted by the original *fakapūlou,* another one may be performed a few days later. In one repeat performance we observed, increased attention was paid to compass directions in the ritual and coconut frond switches *(kahoa, nohoaga)* were incorporated, but the ritual otherwise was essentially the same. The practitioner also chose his plant material from the tops of the tallest trees, rather than from shrubs as he had done on the previous occasion, so that their power would be greater. In this case, both the practitioner himself and the patient's son had been sick after the first *fakapūlou,* circumstances that were believed to indicate the great power of the sorcery.

Several days pass before the final therapeutic ritual in the series. During this time the patient bathes and anoints himself with the prepared oil as he has been directed.

The final ritual, *te fakakaukau* 'the bathing', aims at cleaning the sick person's body of the last vestiges of evil power. A basin of water is prepared and *fetai* vines (*Cassytha filiformis* L.) are scrubbed into it to produce a froth and then removed. Chopped leaves and/or flowers are added, together with coconut oil. The water may have been heated to begin with or red hot axe heads may have been put into it to heat it. In any case, the patient retires to the bathhouse and washes his whole body in the water, putting on clean clothes afterwards. The healer or his assistant then anoints the patient and puts a flower wreath on him.

This should be the end of the problem. If it is not, the washing can be repeated or the whole series performed again. If it seems necessary to repeat the procedures, anointing is prescribed daily in the interval. In deciding how to amend the rituals for the second series, the practitioner might rely on help from a spirit, on his dreams, or on the instructions of the buzzing noise *(ligoligo)* emanating from his bottle of prepared oil.

During the course of treatment the practitioner is himself at risk. The malevolent power may seek to harm him. He is also bound by restrictions that limit his activities. Usually, normal work is forbidden as long as a ritual series is in progress; some practitioners extend this prohibition to the sick person as well, especially to cooking activities for women. It is thus essential for the practitioner to have an assistant who can take care of the heating of the axes, the preparation of materials, and the cleanup afterwards. Care is taken that the ritual implements and also the material residue of the ceremony do not come into contact with anyone, lest they cause injury or death.

The traditional practitioners firmly believe in the morality of the therapy they offer and, in fact, are usually respected and regarded as benevolent by Nanumeans. Over the years the attitude of various pastors toward the practice of power therapies has apparently varied from tacit or outright acceptance to condemnation. During our fieldwork on Nanumea the pastor, himself a Tuvaluan from another island, condemned the practitioners and their therapeutic rituals on the grounds that *vailākau* is the work of the devil. All practitioners are members of the church, however, and they argue that they pray before commencing a therapeutic ritual and when gathering plant material, and that they use their powers only to help people in need. Sick persons who receive therapy are usually Christians, and appear to find no dissonance between the healing rituals and their religious beliefs. One noted Nanumean healer who has traveled on commission to several Pacific countries and to New Zealand to treat illness, explains that from his perspective there is no contradiction between his use of superordinate power and Christianity: the materials which he gathers for his specially treated oil, as well as the oil itself, are all products of God's creation. He is utilizing power which comes from God himself.[17]

In power therapies washing is always a prelude to *teitei* 'anointing'. Similarly, the bathing ritual cleans the patient of the last vestiges of malevolent power by using frothy water in which vines have been scrubbed to create a *hopu mua* (traditional soap). Before any of the ritual sequences are performed, the sick person's house is thoroughly cleaned and all participants, likewise, must first bathe and wear clean clothes. This emphasis on physical/metaphysical cleanliness follows from the ritual's goal of "opening" *(tatala)*[18] the sorcerer's spell so that the evil power can leave (or be driven out of) the patient's body. Once the spell has been opened, the power is washed away and carried off by smoke.

CONCLUSION

Here we would like to comment briefly on some of the general features of Nanumean health beliefs and therapeutic practices that might be particularly relevant to western medical practitioners. These include the relationship between health and strength and its effect on human illnesses, varieties of family support given during illness, and the benefits that derive from having a traditional healing system as a backup to western medical therapies.

Nanumeans equate health with robustness, vitality, and bodily strength. The common positive answer to the question "How are you?" *(E a koe?)* is "Strong, thanks" *(Mālosi, fakafetai)*. Similarly, having a robust body build, neither markedly thin or obese, is believed to indicate health. This implicit connection between strength and health also finds a reflection in the Nanumean attitude that being a "man" is incongruous with being a "sick person." For example, not only are sickly men scorned as "children" *(tamaliki)* but one man with an injured foot that prevented his climbing for drinking nuts commented to us that he felt he "wasn't a man." Though our time-allocation survey showed no marked differences in the time men and women spend incapacitated by illness, Nanumean men clearly find sickness embarrassing. Compared to women and children, they also receive less sympathy while they are ill. Men take conspicuous pride in their ability to perform strenuous male activities like climbing coconut trees, paddling long distances in a canoe, and carrying heavy loads, well into middle and even old age. Because men's work tends to be more physically demanding, illness and injuries can be more disruptive of men's activities than they are of women's.

Even for men, however, sickness is a time for family support. This support typically takes three main forms: physical presence, bodily contact, and feeding. The sick person is believed to benefit from the presence of his kin around him, and the *alofa* 'love, concern, affection' people have for each other is expressed in care *(tausiga)* of the sick. People visit those who are ill and, if needed, often move into the household to help care for them. This sort of support is particularly appropriate when a person is so ill as to move to the hospital compound. It is considered inappropriate and unkind to leave an ill person alone and unattended.

Another valuable form of support in sickness involves bodily contact. The limbs of the sick person, especially the hands, arms, and thighs, are lightly rubbed, stroked, or pressed, often for long periods. Seriously ill infants and young children are held. This physical contact not only relaxes and comforts the patient but also allows those caring for him a tangible way of expressing their concern.

A third main form of support is to indulge and encourage the patient's expression of food whims or cravings. When relatives and neighbours hear of a person's minor illness, they show their sympathy by sending over a delicacy that will tempt the sick person to eat. This might be bread and tea, a kind of fish the person is known to like, a cooked chicken, or, for children, a papaya or cabin crackers. Insofar as food cravings are believed to reflect the physiological needs of the patient's body, catering to them as Nanumeans do should be useful in speeding recovery.

These three forms of support are given relatively easily both in the traditional situation where the sick person is cared for in the household by relatives, and in the village hospital where the patient's household also moves into residence in the hospital compound and continues to care for him or her there. The western hospital milieu, where patients are cared for by medical staff, isolated from their families and expected to eat institutional food, can make it quite difficult for these sorts of support to be provided.

In the case of Nanumea, traditional and western medical therapies combine to form an effective system, one that is best characterized as flexible and pragmatic. Insofar as western medical therapies are available and believed to be effective, people use them. They also use and value traditional therapies. Even though some Nanumeans are skeptical about the efficacy of therapies based on superordinate power, everyone knows of people whom these therapies have apparently helped. Sometimes a "cure" has been effected. In other cases, the process of therapy itself, structured to stretch over several weeks or perhaps even months, provides emotional support and psychological relief. Particularly in the difficult cases that require the repetition of therapeutic rituals, the concern, attention, and expertise directed to securing the sick person's return to health must be both reassuring and gratifying.

The staunchest advocates of the use of traditional therapies are people who have had positive experiences from using them in the past. Their enthusiasm testifies to the continuing ability of traditional healing practices to meet Nanumean needs, an ability that is based on the complementary role they play in relation to an increasingly sophisticated western medical service. Richard Lieban (1973), drawing on Nancie Gonzalez's (1966) work in Guatemala, notes that traditional and western medical therapies may offer "contrastive but complementary gratifications" to the users. The pharmacopoeia of western medicine is usually seen as providing exceptionally effective remedies. Traditional curing therapies, however, offer something else: food and activity prescriptions and avoidances, physical manipulations, and supportive ritual. Traditional therapies also illuminate the ultimate cause believed to lie behind a particular case of illness and thus help to alleviate the psychological stress of being seriously ill. From this point of view, the richness and diversity of Nanumean healing practices make them a cultural asset, worthy of encouragement and preservation.

NOTES

1. This paper is based on field research carried out between May 1973 and January 1975. During that time the authors lived for seventeen months in Nanumea and carried out two months of archival research in Funafuti, Tarawa, and the Western Pacific Archives in Suva. Unless otherwise stated, our comments in this paper refer to Nanumea at the time of that field research.

We are grateful for funding support to the U. S. National Institutes of Health (Training Grant GM 1244) and to the British Overseas Development Administration (U. K. Technical Aid Project No. R2875A & B), Rural Socio-Economic Survey of the Gilbert and Ellice Islands, administered through Victoria University, Wellington.

A number of colleagues have shared information or read and offered comments on an earlier draft of this paper. We wish to thank the Reverend Liu J. Tepou, Ralph Bolton, Michael Goldsmith, Judith Huntsman, Patricia Kinloch, Nancy Lewis, Tom Ludvigson, Doug Munro, and Jay Noricks.

To the people of Nanumea, without whose generous cooperation and hospitality our research would not have been possible, our sincere thanks, *fakafetai lahi kiki*.

2. We use terms such as "local," "indigenous," "traditional," and "western" throughout this paper. In asserting that a practice or belief is local, indigenous, or traditional (these are synonyms in our usage) we are making a distinction that Nanumeans themselves make. When they refer to something as *faka te fenua* 'in the style of the island', they mean something that is believed to be Nanumean, as opposed to "foreign" *(faka pālagi)*. The western-trained doctors, nurses, and dressers in Tuvalu are mostly Tuvaluans, but we have not described their practice of western medicine as local, indigenous, or traditional. Nor is it apparently felt to be so by Nanumeans. We recognize that these western-trained experts may

well respect traditional healing practices, and even patronize traditional healers, but to our knowledge they do not themselves practice both sorts of therapy.

By traditional or indigenous we do not wish to imply that a practice or belief is hoary with age or unchanged since the precontact period. There have been so many changes in Tuvalu culture as a result of contact with Europeans, Samoans, and other peoples that little in the Tuvaluan way of life remains unaffected. Our meaning is simply, as above, that the belief or practice is current today in Nanumea, and is not explicitly seen by people to be alien or in the cultural domain of outsiders.

3. The name Tuvalu, which phonetically is *Tūvalu,* is composed of the morphemes *tū* 'stand' and *valu* 'eight', in reference to the eight permanently inhabited islands in the group. The ninth island—tiny, southernmost Niulakita—was apparently visited for purposes of fowling and turtle hunting, but not regularly inhabited.

4. Details of the events leading up to separation are discussed in Macdonald 1975 and Chambers and Chambers 1975. For the reestablishment of independence see Wilson 1978 and Macdonald 1982, 262ff.

5. Comparable census-based data cited by Macrae 1980 shows that while in Tuvalu, in 1979, male children born alive survived to age two at a rate of 934 per 1000, in Niue this rate was 953 in 1976, and in Fiji (also in 1976) it was 948. For female children survival rates to age two were 947 in Tuvalu, 961 in Niue, and 960 in Fiji. In New Zealand the survival rate for male children to age *one* was 985 per 1000 live births in 1976, and for female children 988 (New Zealand Department of Statistics 1976). In Tuvalu the comparable survival rate to age one was 953 per 1000 for males, and 963 for females (1979 census).

Tuvalu life expectancy at birth can usefully be compared with life expectancies in other Pacific communities. Tuvalu (1973): data for both sexes averaged 54; Tuvalu (1979): males 57, females 60; Niue (1976): males 64, females 64; Western Samoa (1961–66): males 61, females 65; Fiji (1976): males 61, females 64. (All figures from Macrae 1980, 47.) New Zealand life expectancy at birth (1971) was identical to the figure for England and Wales (1969–71): males 69 and females 75 (New Zealand Department of Statistics 1971).

6. Bedford, Macdonald, and Munro 1980 found little written or oral evidence of epidemics or massive disease mortality in postcontact Tuvalu. They conclude from this that the most important effect of these introduced diseases was "some general deterioration in health," and point out that while yaws and filariasis could have debilitating effects, they were "seldom fatal" and usually did not cause the "premature death of an adult." However, they stress that even slight increases in mortality levels, especially among children, can have structural implications for small populations.

Our feeling is that, while mortality from introduced disease may not have been "massive," the recurrent epidemics reported for Tuvalu nonetheless would have had a significant effect on the local population structure. As recently as 1950, for example, forty-five people died in Nanumea in a single year out of a population of 791. Of these deaths, twenty-five were attributed to a "severe influenza epidemic" which afflicted almost the entire population and caused serious pulmonary complications for people over fifty. The epidemic was apparently introduced to Tuvalu by workers returning from employment on Banaba (Gilbert and Ellice Islands Colony 1950).

7. The island served as a staging base for American troops from 1943 to 1945 and some rusting debris was left in the lagoon and offshore shallows. There was also considerable disturbance to reef areas through blasting and dredging. Nanumeans attribute the increase in fish-poisoning cases to the presence of rusting iron and leaking oil. Recent research seems to point to disturbance of reefs as one factor in increased incidence of ciguatera. For a comparative analysis of the severity and frequency of ciguatera fish poisoning and its effect on human health in the island Pacific, see Lewis 1981.

8. Magic, religion, science, and rationality have been topics of classic concern in anthropology since the time of Tylor and Frazer. For recent debate on epistemology, definitions and other issues, see Wax and Wax 1963; Winch 1964; Hammond 1970; Rosengren 1976; and Winkleman 1982.

9. D. G. Kennedy was a teacher, colonial administrator, and amateur ethnographer on the atoll of Vaitupu, Southern Tuvalu, during the 1920s and 1930s. His monograph *Field Notes on the Culture of Vaitupu, Ellice Islands* (1931) is an important source of information on traditional society and culture, as well as on postcontact changes.

10. The phoneme /g/ in Tuvalu is pronounced as the "ng" in English "singer." A macron over a vowel indicates a long vowel. In spoken Nanumean virtually all words with reduplicated syllables of the form "consonant-vowel-consonant-vowel" are pronounced as though the first medial vowel did not exist. This has the effect of lengthening or doubling the consonant. For example, the word written here as *mamae* is pronounced *mmae* in everyday usage. The full reduplicated forms have been written here in deference to Nanumean wishes, and in accord with the policy of the Tuvalu Language Board (1980).

11. The Nanumean language has a limited set of terms for the various concepts which deal with the superordinate realm, and considerable polysemy is found in some words. *Mahaki* 'illness' refers to the more-or-less routine maladies described above. Several descriptive phrases are used to denote illness stemming from the use or misuse of superordinate power. It may be referred to as *mahaki māhei* 'malevolent/evil illness'. Or, one may speak obliquely of the illness as *mea māhei* '[an] evil thing'.

The central concept in this realm is *vailākau,* a term most easily glossed as "medicine," but which has a wide range of other connotations. *Vailākau*, literally "water" + "plant" (or "tree"), can mean a medicinal preparation (herbal, or involving an infusion of coconut oil, leaves, flowers, and possibly grubs), or it can mean a western medicinal substance. *Vailākau*, or its shortened form *vai* 'water', is also the general term for magic as well as sorcery. Thus, to *fakavai* ('cause' + 'water') someone is to place a magic spell on them; to *faivai* ('make' + 'water') is to practice Nanumean medicine. It can also mean to do magic or to manipulate superordinate power. Occasionally the synonym *fai aitu* ('make' + 'spirit') is used instead of *fai vai,* with the meaning "to do magic" or manipulate superordinate power.

A *tagata* (or *tino*) *fai vai* ('man/person' + 'make' + 'water') is a traditional practitioner who may only deal in simple herbal remedies, but who normally would also be versed in healing using rituals which control power from the superordinate realm. A *tagata fai vai māhei* ('man/person' + 'make' + 'water' + 'evil') is a sorcerer.

Jay Noricks (personal communication, Sept. 1982) informs us that on the Tuvalu island of Niutao a distinction is drawn between *tufuga fai masaki* and *tino fai vailākau*. The former specialist treats routine illness while the latter deals with the superordinate realm. Our impression is that Nanumeans do not consistently distinguish terminologically between these two sets of practitioners, and in fact the same person may be adept at both types of therapy.

12. Noricks 1981 discusses aspects of possession and related afflictions for the Tuvalu island of Niutao.

13. None of these simple medicines are sold through the local store; Nanumeans can only obtain them from the medical staff at the island hospital.

14. Our translation here of *te vai e lelei* is but one of several possible. The phrase could also be rendered "the magic is good," or perhaps "the power therapy is good."

15. This bottle is said to be the vehicle for the sorcerer's power and people talk as though it is actually buried under or beside a house post. (Houses generally have earth floors covered with coral pebbles; the massive posts which support the roof structure are dug down a meter or so into the soil and are located inside the living area of the house.) No one seeks to dig up or remove the bottle, however, and its power is nullified through ritual.

16. Iron axes and metal tools in general were introduced to Nanumea during the nineteenth century, replacing adze heads made of *Tridacna* shell. Since the latter cannot withstand heating in fire, and iron implements are relatively recent introductions, the specific procedure described here is either a recent innovation or a recent introduction. Iron axe heads may also be a substitute for hot stones, which may have been used to boil water in precontact times. Even these stones would have had to come from volcanic islands, however.

Kennedy 1931 makes no mention of sorcery as a cause of illness in Vaitupu, nor does he discuss therapeutic rituals of the sort found in Nanumea. The widespread belief in the efficacy of sorcery in Tuvalu today, however, plus the existence of the complex therapies designed to counteract it, suggests the possibility that Kennedy's government position made people reticent to discuss such matters with him.

17. Personal communication from the Rev. Liu J. Tepou, Aug. 1982.

18. It was only in discussing concepts of magic and power with the Rev. Liu J. Tepou during the writing of this paper that some important aspects of the semantics and epistemology of magic fell into place for us. When things or people have been placed under a spell *(fakavai)* they are affected in a manner that leaves them "bound" or "tied" *(hahae)*. They are, in essence, covered up with or closed in by superordinate power *(vai)*. This is seen most explicitly in fishing magic, where through proper exercise of a ritual involving both incantation *(lalau)* and tying knots *(hahae)* an outrigger canoe or fishing net can be made more effective or potent. To do this to a canoe is to *hae vaka* 'knot' or 'tie up' a canoe. Similarly, a specially prepared bottle of coconut oil buried beside a house post "ties up" the

house and its inhabitants (with the result that it makes them ill), and love magic "ties up" or binds the love of the intended victim. The procedures described above for nullifying or counteracting magic are conceived of as "opening" or "unbinding" *(tatala)*. Interestingly, in the case of nets or canoes which are literally, as well as figuratively, knotted, one "opens" the magic by actually cutting away the knots.

3

Healing in Central Espiritu Santo, Vanuatu

Tomas Ludvigson

The following account of healing practices among the Kiai-speaking population of the upper Ari valley in central Espiritu Santo, Vanuatu, is based on seventeen months of social anthropological field research between the years 1974 and 1976.[1]

The Kiai-speaking people live in small, thinly scattered hamlets situated on ridges 500–800 meters above sea level. For subsistence they grow taro and other crops in swidden clearings on the mountainsides, raise pigs and cattle, fish in the streams, and hunt in the forest surrounding the settlements. Despite extensive changes over the last hundred years, they have remained non-Christian and relatively independent of the coastal community and market economy.

To begin with, I discuss diagnosis as it is evident in discussions of illness among local people. After a brief account of the manifestations of illness recognized by my informants, this discussion largely takes the form of an explication of crucial concepts in the several explanatory models employed in interpreting illness. Next I discuss therapies in connection with different types of illness, causation, and healing personnel, whether a local layman or specialist, or someone trained in the western medical tradition. I conclude with a descriptive account of an incident that took place during my fieldwork, showing how the diagnostic and therapeutic models are employed in a real situation of acute illness.

DIAGNOSIS

My access to how the local people diagnose illness was through the talk generated when someone was ill. The terminology they used when talking among themselves about illness revealed to me an array of concepts of processes and existences relevant to both diagnosis and therapy. As my understanding of these indigenous interpretations of illness is so dependent on their speech, I have organized my account around the appropriate Kiai vocabulary.

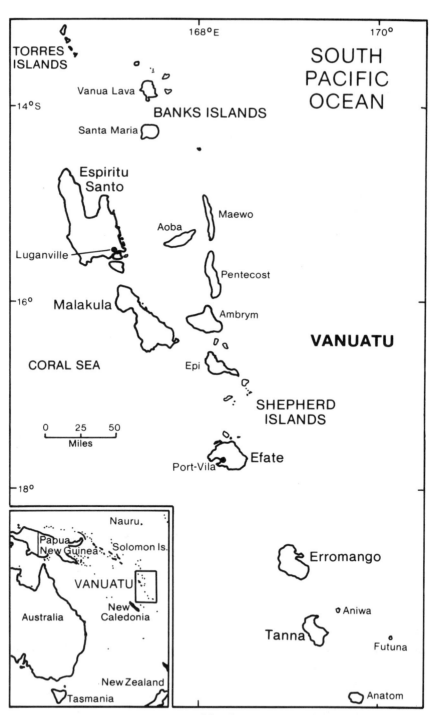

Map 2

Part of that vocabulary refers to illness as it is manifest in experience. Thus, there are words for disorders of bodily function or behavior: *pira* 'have diarrhoea', *sova* 'cough', *ulo* 'vomit', *karum* 'scratch' (as in scabies), *sarsaramariri* 'tremble' (as in malaria), *peropero* 'talk/be crazy', to name but a few. There are words for unhealthy states or conditions of the sick person's body or body part: *varun* 'hot' (as in a fever), *vonovono* 'stopped' (as in constipation), *sosoi* 'swollen', *maloko* 'tired', *mata ara* 'red eye' (as in conjunctivitis), and so on. There are words for pain and sensations associated with illness: *manainas* 'it hurts', *akira* 'feel cold'. There are words for disorders that appear as existences in themselves: *vosa* 'sore', *mezomezo* 'infected sore', *panenainas* 'stomach ache', *patunainas* 'headache'.

The people use these terms when they identify and discuss the particular manner in which a person is ill. Some therapies can be applied at this stage, without further diagnosis. There is, for example, therapeutic magic explicitly directed at headache, stomachache, backache, and the like. Medicines, indigenous or introduced, are also part of immediate therapy.

If this therapy is not successful, and the illness persists or gets worse, diagnosis can be taken a stage further. The illness is then interpreted as a symptom of some underlying cause. This cause must then be attended to (i.e. be removed or nullified) before the illness can come to an end.

Unlike in the western medical tradition, these underlying causes are not systematically related to symptoms in any manner that makes it possible generally to deduce the former from the latter. Instead, the different kinds of causes that are indicated in local discussions of illness seem only loosely connected to the precise manner of being ill.

Diagnostic talk suggests a number of different kinds of causes operating behind illness, individually or in conjunction. I will discuss these causes under the headings of talking spirits, unwholesome food, passion, and sorcery.

Talking Spirits

It is hard to give a brief account of this topic without distorting it. There is not one consistent version, but rather several different and mutually contradictory versions of what is what in the spirit world. These differences in interpretation of phenomena in the realm of spirits are in the main peripheral to their use in the explanation of illness and will not be taken into account here, though I feel that to present only this simplified version and leave out the ambiguities robs the material of much of its vitality—even mystery.[2]

Simply put, spirits cause illness. They strike people with illness by "talking about" them *(vara ini)*. So, for example, when I once had a sudden acute bout of fever the local seer treated me with a charm which he spat into my stomach. He then told me that the spirit of a dead man from a neighboring settlement, which I had just visited before falling ill, had made me ill by talking about me.

The local people are often unclear about what kind of spirit is implicated in any particular instance of illness, and some even maintain that the many words for spirits all refer to the same kind of being. Others speak of different kinds of spirits, and though the spirits all cause illness in the same way, that is, by talking, they are partly differentiated by origin and by the kind of illness they inflict.

The *tamate* are the spirits of the dead. Having abandoned their physical bodies at death, they dwell wild in the forests surrounding the settlements. These spirits rarely afflict adults with disease; children are their chief victims. They can also make people ill by talking about their food.

The *aviriza* are spirits of people killed in feuding in the past. They are said to live on the slopes of two high peaks at the head of the valley. These spirits are described as red. Another name for them is *ape,* though this name is not spoken out loud, as its use is said to attract the spirits, who will strike the speaker with illness.

Though the *aviriza* can cause a variety of complaints, they are particularly implicated in cases of sores *(vosa)* and mental illness *(peropero).* The *aviriza* make people ill by talking, though sometimes a sick person is said to have seen the *aviriza* or to have stepped on their blood, either of these forms of contact being enough to precipitate illness. The *aviriza* can also capture a person's spirit, a form of soul stealing that results in a long coma. Consciousness returns to the victim only when his or her spirit returns.

The *ria* are bush ogres that live in rocks and along watercourses in the bush. They are larger than people and have long arms and legs, tails, and long hair. They are said to eat the people they manage to waylay in the bush at night, though since the advent of firearms on the island the *ria* keep away from the immediate vicinity of the settlements. Some informants say that the *ria* are old people who never died, but just left their homes at an advanced age to live on in the bush.

The *ria* also make people ill, mainly children, by talking about them. Or, while the parents are working in a garden with the little one asleep on some leaves nearby, the *ria* may come close and touch the bedding. In either case the child becomes ill with *zalo i ria* 'ogre sickness', easily recognized by its symptom: the child will *sarsaramariri* 'tremble' with a fever.

Unwholesome Food

Food can cause illness. For example, one of my informants, after a fit of coughing, expressed the concern: "What did I eat today?" And my host in the Ari valley, after hearing me cough, commented to his wife, "Has he eaten *malino*, or what?"

To eat *malino* is to eat unwholesome food. "The sickness is in your stomach," it was explained to me. Coconut milk and coarse trade salt were both foods specifically identified as causing a cough. But any other food can be rendered unwholesome in a variety of ways: (1) by being talked about by a spirit, (2) by an animal's eating part of it (the animal saliva, when ingested, is the cause of the illness), and (3) by age and the processes of putrefaction. Smell *(pona)* is the criterion invoked when people reject food on this last ground.

Passion

Certain actions and emotional states are considered to precipitate illness in the people involved and/or their spouses, children, or other close relatives. The Kiai term for this is *masulu*—to 'catch fire' or 'get hot'.

There are two general areas of application: sexual arousal leading to adultery or extramarital sex, and anger leading to conflict and retaliatory action. This diagnosis is apparent in speculations, allegations, accusations, and confessions of anger and/or sexual intrigue in connection with illness.

For example, when a young boy in a nearby hamlet had an eye infection, a neighbor suggested that the boy's father, absent from the Ari valley while working as a plantation laborer on the South Coast, had found himself a lover there. And after a local man had moved away from the valley because of a quarrel with his neighbors, he told me in private that it was their hard-headedness *(kilan)* that had brought illness on their children. "If you are angry for two or three days, sickness will come," he explained.

The *masulu* mentioned by my informants as precipitating illness was that connected with extramarital sexual play or intercourse in thought, dream, or deed, masturbation, and penile erections. Concerning anger, the *masulu* was said to be manifest in homicide (through violence or sorcery), swearing, and harboring anger.

Sorcery

There are many forms of sorcery; some are prevalent as explanations of illness while others are mentioned only as explanations of death.

Vezeveze are objects charmed by a sorcerer and thrown so as to lodge in the victim's body, causing pains and ultimately death. Typical *vezeveze* are stones, iron nails, bits of wire, or the hard black spikes commonly used as arrow prongs, found in the soft pith of a local tree fern. Whether thrown by hand or shot with bow and arrow, the objects will find their target—landing, for example, on the roof of the house where the unsuspecting victim lies asleep. Then they can be heard as a trickle of running water as they come through the sago thatch and enter the flesh of the intended victim. The person will suffer body pains and be unable to sleep or even lie down comfortably. Unless a seer removes the *vezeveze*, the person will die.

Sasau is sorcery performed on personal leavings, killing the person after a long and debilitating illness. The sorcerer uses a bit of his victim's food, or a piece of a towel or loincloth. I learned about three different methods.

The sorcerer can leave the bit of food in a special *zara i tataui* 'follow place'. I was told that there was no such place in the valley, but the people closer to the South Coast were said to have them.

The sorcerer can tie up the bit of food with string and hang it over a fire. As it dries out and turns black, the victim sickens and dies. My informant called this technique *lizikoro* 'tie dry'.

The sorcerer can cut the top off a tree fern and put the food inside the trunk at the top, then ringbark the tree at the base. As the tree dies and the soft core rots away, the material moves further down inside the trunk, and the victim becomes ill. When the core is gone, leaving only an empty shell, and the bit of food reaches the base of the trunk, the victim dies. This technique is referred to as *kore malavu* 'put tree fern'.

Talk about sorcery performed on personal leavings was not unusual in cases of protracted illness that didn't respond to treatment. And great care was taken to hide our taro peelings after meals taken on the occasional trek to the South Coast, as we passed through the territories of people who were known for their sorcery.

Elioro is another malevolent practice, perhaps best described as contact sorcery. The sorcerer buries a deadly object in such a place that the intended victim or victims come into contact with it, with illness and death as a result. A charmed kava root *(Piper methysticum)*, or a bamboo tube filled with blood (e.g. lizard's blood or menstrual blood), is a deadly object. It can be buried on a path where the intended victim walks, or under a person's mat at his or her habitual sleeping place inside a house, or at the source of a stream of drinking water. I heard several tales of *elioro* killings in both the remote and recent past, but no illness or death during my fieldwork was attributed to these techniques.

Papa is soul stealing. The sorcerer has a hole in the ground into which he calls the name of his victim. The soul of the victim leaves his or her body and answers back from inside the hole. It remains trapped there, unable to return to its body, which remains unconscious until death. This form of sorcery is said to have come to an end in my field area. The last old man known for *papa* died during my time there, with no one to continue the practice. I never heard *papa* sorcery used as an explanation of any particular case of illness or death.

Sui 'bone' refers to rape sorcery. With the aid of a charmed human bone the sorcerer makes himself invisible, enters a house where a woman lies asleep, and has sexual intercourse with her without her knowing. *Sui* sorcery brings illness through passion—even the sorcerer himself is endangered by his clandestine activities. So, when a young man in a neighboring village was ill for a protracted period, one of the many interpretations of his plight was that he had *sui* and was suffering the consequences of his extramarital sexual affairs.

Patua is a form of assault sorcery. The sorcerer has two little spirit children *(patua)*, invisible to others, who come to him when he is asleep. The *patua* want liver and entrails to eat, and will go hunting with their master. Together with his spirit they enter a house where someone is asleep and cut open his stomach. After the *patua* have eaten the victim's insides, they stuff the cavity with leaves and seal up the wound so that it does not show. In the morning there is no trace of the operation, but the victim will be dead within a day.

The spirit of a sorcerer out hunting with his *patua* will assume the form of an owl, or a fowl, dog, or cat. As such it is vulnerable, and can be killed by killing the animal in question. Then the sorcerer will die within a day.

Though *patua* were never implicated in the case of illness, there was rarely a death without *patua* talk being generated. Generally, the deceased person was seen to be a victim of *patua* sorcery, though in some cases the deceased was said to have been shot in animal form while out hunting with his *patua*.

THERAPY

There is a multitude of paths leading from illness to recovery in central Santo. Some involve consulting a specialist, whether a local seer *(kleva)* or a paramedic *(dresa)* or other practitioner trained in western medicine. Some rely on knowledge of practices more generally distributed among the population. Others are spontaneous and require no conscious strategy or application. I will discuss them in turn under the headings of medicines, magic, dieting, and disclosure.

Medicines

The forest and gardens surrounding the settlement yield many different varieties of plant material for the preparation of medicines. For internal use by the ill person there are leaves to chew and drinks made from ground roots or bark. Leaves are also applied externally, to sores and swellings, sometimes after first being rendered into a paste by mastication.

When I was stricken with dysentery during an extended visit to a hamlet on the far side of the valley, for example, a local man brought me leaves to chew twice a day for two days. When I asked him what leaves he was using, he took me to a large mountain-apple tree *(Eugenia malaccensis)* nearby and showed me the procedure: pick some leaves and tear each of them in two along the stem down the middle, throwing away one half and keeping the other. Then make sure that you have an even number of half-leaves—two, four, six, eight, or ten. It doesn't matter how many, as long as the half-leaves all form pairs. Roll them up together and they are ready to be chewed. My informant and would-be healer told me that the leaves were effective against both diarrhoea and cough.

Knowledge of such remedies is widespread and freely imparted. They are supposed to be effective in themselves, and need not be accompanied by any magical charms. They can be prepared and administered by anybody who knows how to, including the ill person.

At the time of my fieldwork, medicines imported from metropolitan countries were made available to the local people from several different outlets. A western pharmacy a well as many Chinese stores in the township of Luganville sell simple medicines such as aspirin and various creams and ointments. Coastal dispensaries and a French hospital at Luganville are occasionally consulted by mountain people, but usually only as a last resort after other therapies have failed to produce the desired result. More frequently, the local people take their ailing children to one of two "dressers"—Melanesian paramedics stationed as part of the British public health service in Waylapa village on the South Coast and in the mission village of Tombet in the northern interior. The Tombet dresser also made house calls on request all over the mountainous center of the island, dispensing ointments, pills, and syrups, dressing sores, and giving injections. Having had some medical training, I did the same throughout my own stay in the Santo mountains.

Magic

As elsewhere in Melanesia, there is magic intended for a variety of purposes, not all of them concerned with healing. There is, for example, magic to bring rain or sunshine, growth magic for pigs and crops, and magic to ward off hurricanes, as well as love magic, magic to cause illness (as in the kinds of sorcery mentioned above), and magic to repel an unwanted suitor.

Magic is known as *maumau* in Kiai. Common to all magic is a verbal formula *(vete)*, spoken or silently recited by the magician, and then somehow transmitted to its object. Some magic is spat directly into the body of the patient. Some is spat into water or other kinds of drink, or onto leaves to be chewed or rubbed on the patient's body. Some is directed not at the body of the patient but at the *aviriza* thought to have captured his or her spirit. This magic is then spat onto a bamboo tube which is blown as a trumpet in the direction of the high peaks at the head of the valley where the *aviriza* are said to live.

Most of the ordinary, everyday performances of therapeutic magic take place unheralded, when called for, in people's homes. Consequently, I had my most intimate views of these practices when I was the patient myself. Once when I fell ill, for example, vomiting with a high fever and lying incapacitated on my sleeping mat for more than twenty-four hours of continuous agony, the local seer came to me with an offer to treat my condition.

He squatted beside my mat and told me to sit up. I propped myself up with arms behind my back. He reached out and started scratching at the sides of my abdomen with short, quick movements of his hands while looking absently to the side. Then he made a semicircular movement with his hands, starting at my sides and bringing his thumbs together at my solar plexus, where he pressed hard, while spitting a few times at my stomach. He went through the same performance three times in a row. "The spirit of a dead man at Zinoi made you ill," he told me when I asked him what he had done. The spirit had talked about me.

Magic is traditional, passed down through the generations. Most adult men know some, but certain old men are credited with greater knowledge due to their longer life. They are sometimes visited by relatives with sick children to be healed. One of them explained to me the interplay between diagnosis and therapy. He knew many magical formulae. "You try one," he said. "If it does not work you try another. You keep trying different ones until you hit on the right formula for the illness in question. Then it ends at once."

A few people learned their magical charms from spirits. These people are known as *kleva,* or *matalesi*—literally, "see-eye." They are seers, supposedly able to "see" directly the causes of illnesses. It was explained to me that this gives them an advantage over other healers: because of their superior diagnostic powers, their therapy is less a matter of trial and error and they always know which charms to use for each condition.

Although these diagnostic powers are commonly understood as a direct seeing of the cause of illness, the one seer with whom I discussed this matter explained it differently. He had been sought out by a spirit in the form of a lizard, which now came to him at night and imparted to him knowledge of the causes of particular cases of illness in the community along with instructions on what leaves and formulae to use to treat them.

One of the seers told me about his practice when fetched to another village to treat an ill person:

It works like this. I go, I pronounce the cause, and the illness ends. Then I go and fetch leaves for it. When I return I charm them. Then I give them to the ill person and he hits his body with them. He singes them in a fire, he uses them, and then the illness ends.

He just applies heat to his heart. He is cold through to his fingers and all over. He is cold, as if his blood doesn't run—like it is still, and he is dying.

I take the leaves, I hold them against his chest, making his heart warm again, making his whole body so that his blood starts running again under his skin, and he gets well. The leaf just turns to ashes.

The seers are the only healers to use a therapeutic technique called *avuavuti* 'pull out'. I saw a seer do this at Tonsiki on the far side of the valley. Squatting next to his patient, he picked up two large leaves in each hand. Then, holding the leaves flat against each hand with a thumb, he placed them next to each other on his patient's shoulder, pulling them down her arm and bringing them together in one movement, finally folding up the leaves and tucking them under the toes of his left foot. He repeated the treatment on the woman's other arm, legs, and back.

Another seer explained to me that when they *avuavuti*, they pull out "bits of rat food, bits of lizard food. They remove the things that are making the person ill—like blood, but it isn't blood. Like the spit of some bad thing that lives on the ground. Then the man's body gets well again."

Some seers were said to be able to remove *vezeveze* objects and produce them for an astonished audience to admire. I never saw this feat performed during my stay in the Santo mountains, but I was told of instances when informants had seen it done.

Dieting

It is common to follow magical therapy with a restricted diet, spoken of as a *tapu* on eating certain foods. The restriction applies to the person who has been treated with magic, but in the case of a child's illness it is extended to his or her parents. Typical foods restricted in such dieting are coconuts, prawns, fish, cane shoots *(Saccharum edule),* and island cabbage *(Hibiscus abelmoschus).*

I was never given an explanation of why certain foods should be avoided after *maumau* beyond the idea that it was a necessary condition for the therapy to remain effective. Or, in the words of a local seer:

A man fetches a leaf. He takes his leaf and says, "This is my leaf. If you eat it and get well, your *tapu* will be to not eat these things." Like you don't eat prawns, or you don't eat coconuts. This means that you will stay well for a long time, like it will be two or three years before you get ill again. But if you eat it soon again, then you will become ill again. It works just like that. That's all there is to it.

Disclosure

The therapy that counters the sickness-inducing effects of passion is confession. Because passion can cause illness both in the "hot" *(masulu)* person and in his or her spouse, child, or other close relative, it is always ambiguous whether it is the patient or someone else who is the guilty party needing to confess in order to bring the illness to an end.

When the patient confesses, it is called *vavaulu* 'to confess'. When a close relative of the patient confesses, this is referred to as *vavaulu isina* 'confess to him/her': the guilty party reveals to the ill person the hidden passion seen to be a probable cause of the illness.

One informant explained to me that if people do not confess, the magical therapy does not work. So, if after *maumau* the patient has not improved, the implication would be that some passion remains unconfessed. For example, when a young Zinoi seer remained ill for a long time, despite both magical therapy and a week at the French hospital in Luganville, one informant suggested that it was because the sick man had *vanu tei* 'bad things'. My informant then told me his reasons for believing that the sick man had used rape sorcery. It was the undisclosed extramarital sex that was the cause of the illness, he suggested, as the sick man would not confess out of fear of the husbands of the many women he had raped. In such a situation treatment may be withdrawn. As another informant put it, "Who's going to tire himself out making magic when they don't confess?"

Confession can be seen as part of a broader theme involving secrecy and disclosure. Generally, it appears that secrecy is a condition for the effectiveness of the various influences behind illness, and to disclose a hidden cause renders it powerless.

We can detect this notion at work in some of the preceding therapies. In the seer's own explanation of his procedure, quoted in the discussion of magic, the disclosure of the cause ends the illness, and the subsequent therapy merely serves to bring the patient's body back to a healthy state. Also, the magical formulae for healing spirit-induced illness contain lists of names of individual *tamate* or *aviriza,* or of places known to be haunted by *ria*. The magic works through naming correctly the spirit responsible.

Another instance is the idea that an ill person will recover spontaneously after seeing the cause of his plight in a dream, such as a rat stealing a bit of his food, or the spirit of a dead person.

A REAL-LIFE SITUATION

I have organized the preceding discussion under the headings of diagnosis and therapy. This distinction is somewhat artificial, as it obscures the interplay, or mutual dependence, between the two types of activity in real-life situations of illness. For example, diagnosis is hard to distinguish from therapy when disclosure of the cause of an illness is itself considered therapeutic, as we have seen above. Also, therapy is often itself a part of the diagnostic process, when the success or failure of a particular therapy (taken to be always effective against a certain kind of illness or cause) reveals whether or not the diagnosis was correct, and so informs subsequent diagnosis.

It is appropriate to emphasize here that the diagnostic and therapeutic models outlined above are of my own construction. They are hypotheses formulated to make sense of how the Kiai-speakers address illness in word and deed. The people did not themselves systematize their knowledge about illness and healing in this fashion. Instead, what they said often seemed partial, haphazard, even contradictory—at least to me, brought up in a tradition of systematic accounts.

In order to remedy this analytic bias, I conclude by relating an incident from my time in the Ari valley. It concerns something as everyday as a small girl having an attack of what I took to be malaria, which was endemic in my field area. This account will, I hope, balance my systematic presentation with a glimpse of the contingent, if not chaotic, way in which diagnosis and therapy take place in a real situation.

I happened to be working on my fieldnotes at a table in front of the house I shared with a local family when a call from my hostess, Veaki, brought me back to the present. I left my books on the table, stood up, and went inside to see what was the matter.

There were many people inside, mostly women with small children. They had stayed behind talking to Veaki after a festive meal of mashed five-leaf yam pudding with coconut milk. In the light from the back entrance I could make out some of them seated by the still-warm oven stones in the rear of the house.

Veaki directed me over to where Noti Lepa from Patunvonara was sitting in the shadows halfway along the wall on my right, her second-youngest daughter on her lap. Old Mala, squatting beside her, held the girl around the waist in a firm, two-handed grip, halfway through some therapeutic magical formula. The girl had just vomited in the course of an attack of fever. There was a note of panic in her mother's voice as she told me about it.

I could understand Noti Lepa's distress—the girl felt very hot to the touch. I took her hand and felt for her pulse with the tips of my fingers. It was incredibly fast. Looking down at my wristwatch, I counted sixty beats in fifteen seconds. I could hardly believe it. How could she survive a pulse rate of two hundred and forty? I looked at the girl, half expecting her to pass away before my very eyes.

It was probably malaria. Earlier that same day Noti Lepa had brought the girl to me, saying that she had become ill with a fever every day shortly before noon. I had given her two chloroquine tablets, but not in time to prevent one last, violent attack of ague. If my diagnosis was correct, the girl would be all right tomorrow—the antimalarials never failed to do the job. But would she make it through another day? Would her barely three-year-old body stand up to the strain of that fever?

I hesitated. I had been called inside to help, but there was not much I could do. All I could think of was something to get the fever down, though the seeming futility of salicylic acid as a lifesaver only increased my all-too-familiar feeling of helplessness in the face of acute illness. Still, I put some water in the bottom of an enamel cup, added half a tablet of soluble aspirin, and pushed my way through the small crowd now surrounding Noti Lepa and the girl.

Mala had finished his *maumau*. Now it was Merei Aki, the girl's father, who was repeating what seemed to me essentially the same procedure—the grip around the waist, the intermittent spitting. I gave the cup of dissolved aspirin to Noti Lepa, who promptly lifted it to her lips and drained it, then bent over and sprayed the contents into the mouth of her barely conscious daughter.

Finished with my own contribution, I got out of the way, content to watch the growing commotion from my nearby mat. The news had spread, shouted, to Moropaka, and more people kept coming into the house all the time, adding to the confusion. The din rose with the many questions of the curious and the agitated explanations of those in the know. Within minutes the house was crowded. In the midst of all the turmoil I saw Sari sip water from a cup and blow clouds of spray at the girl from different directions. Next Soro, just arrived from Moropaka, followed Mala and Merei Aki with still another stomach-pressing bout of *maumau*.

"The medicine struck her," suggested a voice in the ongoing proceedings. By now it was common knowledge that I had given the girl some pills that morning.

"No," retorted Mala. The cause was a long-standing quarrel between neighbors that had threatened to flare up again that morning. A child had returned home to Moropaka after playing at Lotuaroi, bearing the tale that Noti Lepa had brought the quarrel to my host, Sari. As one of our chief's assistants, Sari was used to being approached by people with a grievance, as a first step towards formal settlement of the matter through arbitration.

Noti Lepa denied reporting anything to Sari, though in fact I had heard her talk to him about the quarrel when she came to Lotuaroi for medicine that morning. The child must have overheard her. Now she took a different attitude. If the quarreling continued, they—herself, Merei Aki, and their six children—would move away and settle somewhere else, by themselves.

Next she launched into an extended monologue, pouring out antipathy for the neighboring couple with whom she and her husband had been quarreling. She spoke at length, describing the quarrel in detail and occasionally addressing her neighbors with rhetorical questions as if they were present—a practice I had noted in angry men's speeches by the kava bowl. Never again were they to use Merei Aki's shotgun. Never again were they to bring their sick children to Merei Aki for *maumau*.

There was an occasional comment or question about details in her angry lament, but for the most part she spoke without interruption. Eventually Noti Lepa came to the end of her tirade and calmed down, and the talk again became more general, with others offering their opinions on the situation. Sari's comment, filled with foreboding, brought home to me the broader significance of the situation as it affected the whole community: "Feet of anger are treading about. When the place is hot like that, days of sickness will come."

Eventually the crowd dispersed. Most of them went to eat at a nearby house. They had just opened up an oven there and put out a call for all to come and eat more yam pudding.

I went over to Noti Lepa and took her daughter's pulse again. It had dropped to one hundred and eighty, and I told Noti Lepa that the girl would be all right.

"Yes," said Noti Lepa. It was because she had *vavaulu isina* 'confessed to her'. I hadn't realized that this was what her long monologue had been about! Noti Lepa had confessed her anger, the ostensible source of her daughter's illness. And—predictably?—the girl was already better.

NOTES

1. My research was generously funded by Stiftelsen Lars Hiertas Minne (The Lars Hierta Memorial Foundation), Statens Rad For Samhallsforskning (The Swedish National Council for Social Research), and the Auckland University Research Committee.

2. A less one-dimensional account of this material can be found in my Ph.D. thesis, "Klevā: Some Healers in Central Espiritu Santo, Vanuatu," University of Auckland, 1981.

4

Contemporary Healing Practices in Tikopia, Solomon Islands

Judith Macdonald

This chapter, based on fifteen months' fieldwork during 1979–80, discusses the contemporary healing beliefs and practices in Tikopia, a small Polynesian outlier in the eastern part of the predominantly Melanesian Solomon Islands. Santa Cruz, the nearest island with a doctor and a small hospital, and main island of the Eastern Outer Islands Province, is two hundred fifty miles away. Honiara, the capital of the Solomons and the location of the major hospital, is six hundred miles to the west. The only means of transport between Tikopia and the rest of the Solomons are the ships which now call about once a month.

Tikopia's size and isolation inhibited frequent contact with the outside world for a long time. The first recorded visit to Tikopia by Europeans was by Quiros in 1606 but apparently no further outside contact was made for another two hundred years. During the nineteenth century, explorers, whalers, and labor recruiters visited the island, and at the beginning of the twentieth century the Church of Melanesia first put mission teachers on Tikopia (Firth 1959, 31–41). In 1980 approximately twelve hundred people lived on the island, which is 3.5 km long and 2 km at its widest part. A freshwater lake takes up about a quarter of the area, leaving enough land for the production of ample food for subsistence but no surpluses that could be used for commercial purposes, such as the production of copra. The lack of exploitable commodities, combined with a small population from which relatively few men can be spared as wage laborers, has helped to maintain a way of life not now seen in most parts of Oceania.

Visits to the island by anthropologists over the last fifty years have produced a record of slow change. Raymond Firth, who first worked among the Tikopians in 1928–29, has written extensively about the people and their beliefs before the island had been completely converted to Christianity.[1] At the time of his first visit he found that approximately half the population and three of the four *ariki* 'chiefs' retained belief in

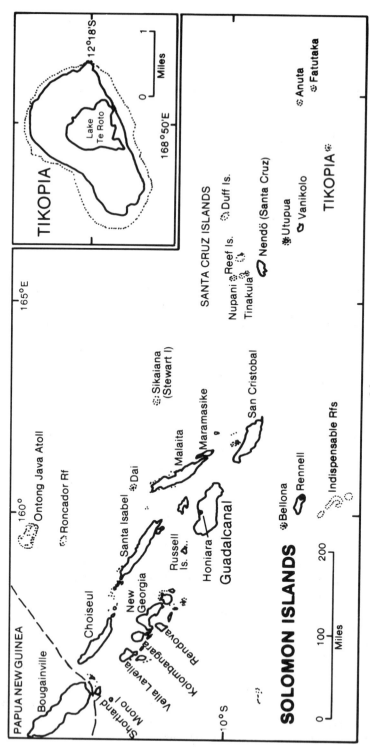

Map 3

their indigenous gods and spirits and conducted ceremonies and rites to influence them (Firth 1970, 305). Beliefs about sickness and healing, as will be discussed later, were part of the traditional spiritual schema.

Firth, with James Spillius, returned to Tikopia in 1952. Spillius remained there for eighteen months, during a time of famine and crisis following two cyclones and an influenza epidemic. To relieve pressure on the scarce and slowly regenerating resources, men were encouraged to leave Tikopia and settle as copra workers on a Lever Brothers plantation in the Russell Islands. Although a few Tikopian men had gone away to other parts of the Solomons previously, it was only with this organized scheme that significant numbers began to leave, and later return to, the home island.[2] In 1966 Firth made a third, brief visit to Tikopia and found that it was by then completely converted to Christianity and that the spirit mediums, intermediaries between men and spirits who had been active in the diagnosis and relief of illness during his previous visits, were no longer practicing. This was, in part, due to the interdict against spirit mediums by the church to which all Tikopians in 1965 nominally belonged. Only the Church of Melanesia, as the Church of England is known in this area, had established itself on the island and the spiritual welfare of the people was entirely in the hands of the Anglican priest and his catechists. Earlier in the century the functionaries of the church had been Melanesians, but by 1980 the priest and his assistants were Tikopian.

At the time my fieldwork was carried out, Tikopians had been traveling freely to and from other islands for almost thirty years with the concomitant introduction of new ideas, new diseases, and new remedies. Some medical aid was available in Tikopia, the church was apparently firmly established, and a few spirit mediums had resumed their practice.

In this description of contemporary healing practices in Tikopia I intend to show how several different approaches to sickness and its alleviation have been combined. It begins with a European analysis of the state of health on the island, followed by a brief summary of the social organization and its relevance to health. The body of the discussion deals with the recognition of certain maladies and the response to them, as well as the presentation of illustrative case studies.

A EUROPEAN VIEW OF HEALTH IN TIKOPIA

In 1980 the Tikopians appeared to be a healthy and physically fit group of people. They are lean but well-muscled and few of them carry any spare fat; most are able to climb to their gardens on the mountainsides until quite an advanced age. Their teeth are black from chewing betel nut but few people have missing teeth unless they have spent some time on other islands where sugar is available. My impression of their fitness was confirmed by Dr. J. Norwood, a medical practitioner attached to the Santa Cruz hospital in 1980, whose job it was to look after the health of the Eastern Outer Islands Province. Dr. Norwood said that the Tikopians, with their well-balanced diet, which includes plenty of fish, are at an advantage compared with some of their neighbors whose diet appears to be more limited.

The male nurse at the clinic on Tikopia said that there is no heart disease or circulatory problems such as varicose veins or hemorrhoids. The greatest number of complaints treated at the clinic involved, in adults, skin diseases and wounds; in children, chest infections and diarrhoea. Five of the eight parishes on the island have kept incomplete registers of births, deaths, and marriages over the last six years, but it is impossible to make generalizations about life expectancy from such limited information. The nurse suggested that the majority of deaths were those of babies under about three months who died of chest infections such as pneumonia and bronchitis, and old people who died of being old. A rough estimate made from the Solomon Islands Census of Population, 1976, shows that 3 percent of the Tikopian population is over the age of seventy compared with less than 1 percent in the Melanesian group. The few deaths in the middle-age range were usually caused by accidents such as drowning or falling from trees and cliffs.

From contact with other parts of the Solomons, tuberculosis has been introduced and, although malaria is not endemic to the island, some migrant Tikopians have contracted it. It was also suggested by the nurse that some men are returning with venereal disease and liver damage from alcohol, which is available elsewhere but not in Tikopia.

While the Tikopians have words which mean "clean" and "dirty," these terms are simply descriptive of visible appearance, except for those Tikopians who have had extended contact (through paramedical training, for example) with European ideas about transmission of disease. Having no germ theory of disease, the Tikopians do not take steps to avoid contamination of food by flies or dirt; a piece of food dropped on the ground has the visible dirt brushed off and is eaten. Equally, despite the nurse's attempts at education in western ways of thinking about hygiene, there appears to be no idea of avoiding contact with those who have skin complaints, and pipes and wads of chewed betel nut may be exchanged with people suffering from tuberculosis. Virtually every adult on the island chews betel nut; its distribution is part of each ceremonial occasion and it is the accompaniment to everyday work and leisure. The chewing of betel nut stimulates salivation and necessitates copious expectoration, so it is common to see men, from their position in the center of the house, spitting, with varying degrees of accuracy, long streams of betel juice toward the low doorway through which the only access to the house is on hands and knees. While the Tikopians bathe at least twice a day, they do not wash their hands before preparing food or eating.

The people tend to urinate at the side of the path or near houses. On one side of the island they go into the sea to defecate, but on the other side the lake is used for this purpose as well as for bathing and washing clothes. After a prolonged dry spell the lake water near the villages visibly effervesces with bacterial action. Drinking water, recently piped into each village, comes from springs high on the mountain and above a level at which it might become polluted.

It is apparent that western concepts of hygiene and transmission of disease are neither understood nor practiced by the majority of Tikopians despite the attempts of the nurse and schoolteachers to inculcate them.

TIKOPIAN IDEAS ABOUT ORDER AND HEALTH

Tikopia is a hierarchically stratified society. Four *ariki* 'chiefs' are the hereditary heads of four clans, each helped in the administration of his clan by the senior men of each lineage who can be seen as executive officers. (Formerly, the elders of the traditional ritual cycle held important positions in the community, but they have now been supplanted by the Christian priest.) The commoners form the largest part of a community in which men have authority over women. A similar hierarchical structure is seen in the formation of groups: all Tikopians belong to the *kano-fenua* 'whole land'; then to smaller groups, namely the clan, the lineage, and the household. Office holders or senior men at each level have a commensurate degree of *mana* 'power', which can be used to bless or to curse. The *ariki,* at the top of the hierarchy, and most powerful of all, are believed to have the power to cause fatal illness in someone who has offended them, or conversely, to stave off death or cause life to begin with the touch of their hands.

Ideas about the political and social order of the land are often expressed in metaphorical statements about the body and its well-being. For example, it is believed that "the body of the chief is the body of the land." An aged and decrepit *ariki* is thought to mean that the land will bear poorly, reflecting the lack of vigor of its chief. It is also said that if two groups of people from one clan fight, it is as if the body is fighting itself and the *ariki,* symbolic body of his clan, will become sick. Then, not only will the fighting parts of the clan suffer, but the clan as a whole. The idea that a malfunctioning part undermines the welfare of the whole is extended to each level of the hierarchy. Hence, a woman who commits adultery will cause sickness to members of her household, either her husband or her child.

Social disorder brings misfortune in the shape of sickness, sterility of land and people, or other disasters. The remedy therefore is to restore order by resolving a quarrel, by confession and apology or, in the case of extreme recalcitrance, the *ariki* may expel an offender from the land.

The idea of "inside" and "outside" is one that is both implicit and explicit in the worldview of many island communities. "Inside" is the bounded physical world of the island and its social organization; "outside" are the foreigners who live across the sea. In some circumstances the spirit realm is also regarded as being a foreign domain. As the order of the land can be disturbed by internal pressures, it can also be disrupted by intrusions from outside. Inhabitants of the spirit world may interfere in human lives, causing sickness or death, and contact with non-Tikopians can also produce undesirable consequences. A Tikopian song (Firth 1936, 36) recognizes the danger:

> We here, great is the greed of our eyes
> For the valuables from abroad
> Which come with disaster.

SICKNESS AND HEALING

This section deals with different types of sickness and the Tikopians' response to them. The generic term for sickness is *ngaengae,* which can be glossed as either "sick" or "sickness." *Ngae* alone can mean "weak." *Ngaengae* is used to indicate fatigue and disinclination for company as well as physical derangement; malaise as well as disease. A complaint of illness raises questions designed to elicit more detail—for example, "Where are you sick?" The reply *ngaengae fuarei,* "just sick," can be taken to mean that the respondent is tired, embarrassed, angry, or in some other state in which he is not predisposed to being sociable. Other responses can be descriptive of a specific symptom, *toku tua e isu,* "my back is sore"; or a general statement of cause, *te toto pariki,* literally "the bad blood," said by a woman with menstrual cramps.

One way of describing the process of sickness alleviation is by identification of symptoms, followed by a diagnosis of their cause and the prescription of a remedy. This model is of limited use in Tikopia where, in some cases, diagnosis may precede symptom by some years. In fact, no one model, either imposed or indigenous, covers the variety of strategies used by the Tikopians to resolve sickness (although at another level the idea of social disruption causing misfortune has some explanatory value). Symptomatology and etiology are not necessarily connected and the only consistency in the therapies used is their intention to restore *maroro* 'health' and relieve discomfort.

For ease of discussion I will divide responses to sickness into three categories which are not necessarily discrete. The Tikopians use certain descriptive phrases when they talk about sickness which suggested these categories to me, but they themselves do not necessarily see sickness this way. The categories are (1) *te ngaengae fuarei* 'just sickness', (2) sickness and cure from outside, and (3) *fakafuaa* 'bringing sickness by spirit means'. Categories 1 and 3 can be seen as a division between those complaints identified by symptoms and those identified by cause. Category 2 contains introduced sickness which may be identified in either manner.

Te Ngaengae Fuarei *'Just Sickness'*

The Tikopians recognize that certain afflictions, usually identified by their symptoms, simply occur and will later disappear, either without treatment or after the application of practical remedies. The term *ngaengae* is not applied to all of them (for example, hiccups) while others which are called *ngaengae* are more distemper of the spirit. A description of some of them and the therapies used is given below.

Hiccups *(tokomauri)* in infants are treated by pasting a piece of *raupita* (betel creeper leaf) to the child's diaphragm with saliva. If the child is very young it is thought that its afterbirth is not buried firmly enough and someone will go to stamp down the ground over it.

Eye irritations and infections are recognized. A discharging eye in babies is irrigated with breast milk while styes and conjunctivitis are treated with juice squeezed from the leaf stem of the *nonu* tree *(Morinda citrifolia)*.[3]

An upset stomach, diarrhoea *(fetiri,* lit. "runs") and dysentery *(tiko toto,* lit. "blood excretion") are all treated with different types of food. Cooked taro left to become moldy, cooked green pawpaw, and the scum from the surface of the water in which rice has been boiled are all used.

There are several different terms for different types of skin complaint, although increasingly the pidgin English word *bakua* is used to refer to most skin disturbances. The Tikopians use the following terms: *fakafoa* or *kufa* 'boil or swelling', *fune* 'scabies', *kaifaariki* or *para* 'ringworm', *maranga* 'spots or prickly heat', *mangeo* or *tona* 'yaws or ulcerations'. Smaller patches of ringworm are sometimes burned out with lime (from burnt coral), a traditional remedy. Today, however, most sufferers go to the clinic where antifungicides are available. In addition, travelers returning from other parts of the Solomons bring back patent remedies for these very common complaints. More serious skin complaints involving persistent ulceration are invariably treated at the clinic with injections of penicillin or another antibiotic.

Cuts *(pakia)* are treated by chewing a very young coconut leaf to a paste and plastering it across the cut to stop bleeding.

Sprains *(makuku)* and broken bones are treated by people, usually men, who are believed to be particularly skillful in this area. One report recalls an instance when a man was called from another district to treat a teenage boy who had slipped on some rocks and sprained his ankle. The man asked the boy's mother to heat an oven stone which was wrapped in layers of barkcloth to make it bearable to the touch. He then gently rubbed the leg and the injured ankle for a few minutes and pressed the hot stone about the swollen part, alternating massage and pressure for about half an hour. Each morning for four days he returned to repeat the treatment. This man was well known for his ability to treat bone and joint injuries, and a European doctor had complimented him on his successful setting of a broken elbow.

While treatment of injury to the skeleton and its points of articulation was carried out by a specialist using massage and heat, massage *(toroi)* alone was used for many other complaints. Tired or sore muscles and the painful stomach accompanying digestive upsets were also treated with massage, but these cases were not ones for specialists. Every adult was capable of administering massage but there were certain social restrictions on who could massage whom. A chief might gently stroke the body of a high-ranking man who was ill, the treatment in this case lying more in the spiritual power *(mana)* of the *ariki* than in the physical manipulation. A married woman could treat her husband, but on the whole it was a service performed for another of the same sex and similar status. For instance, a son would be reluctant to massage his father because of the respectful avoidance required in this relationship.

On three occasions I was treated with massage by women from my neighborhood: once for a strained back, once for a fever with aching joints, and once for general unhappiness and homesickness. In each case the technique was to rub the arms and legs and bonier parts of the body quite gently and to pinch the fattier areas such as the buttocks rather firmly. In cases of *ngaengae* which were tiredness or unhappiness rather than sickness, massage was sometimes offered as a friendly and comforting gesture unless the sufferer pulled a sheet over his head to show he was asleep, or he wished to be regarded as such, in which case he was left alone.

Leaves (*rau rakau,* lit. "tree leaf") were used therapeutically in several ways. The juice of leaves and leaf poultices have already been mentioned. Infusions of cetain broken or chopped leaves were taken for diarrhoea, constipation, and coughs. It appears that one type of leaf is used for one complaint, and I was not given any of the complicated herbal recipes compounded of many ingredients that are common in some other parts of Polynesia.

Sickness from Outside

The history of European contact with the previously isolated island communities of Oceania is a record of devastating epidemics. Complaints such as colds that affected Europeans mildly proved serious or even fatal in communities unused to them. By the time Firth carried out his initial fieldwork in 1928–29 the Tikopians had become aware that new diseases were being introduced to the island.

> From time to time epidemics occur, brought, as the natives themselves realize clearly, by foreign vessels. The generic native term for epidemic disease is *maki* or *makimaki,* and they distinguish such types as *tare,* cough or common cold, *tiko toto,* blood excretion (dysentery). Measles, influenza and other complaints have been introduced in this way, and usually rage with extreme virulence. . . . The Tikopia, ignorant of the germ theory of disease, believe that an epidemic is due to the malignancy of those in control of the vessel. They associate it also to some extent with the blowing of the ship's whistle, so that the captain of the *Southern Cross,* at their request, abstained from the usual practice when weighing anchor. The onset and disappearance of a wave of common colds which followed the visit of the ship when I was set down on the island was a perfect illustration of the spread of an infection. It was gone in about a month, and did not recur during my whole stay. To the rarity of calls of ships from the outside world is largely due the maintenance of the splendid health of this physically fine people. (Firth 1936, 413)

Southern Cross was the ship of the Melanesian Mission, and Firth also notes that many disasters such as hurricane, drought, and epidemic were blamed on the malevolence of a missionary bishop (1936, 36). The mission ship was one of the few vessels to call at Tikopia in the early part of this century and its visits were infrequent, possibly only once a year. Under these circumstances it was not surprising to find outbreaks of epidemic disease. Tyrrell describes the effect of ships calling on similarly isolated communities (1977, 137–44). It was surprising, however, to find that outbreaks of colds still followed the arrival of a ship, although by 1980 that was an almost monthly occurrence. People called it *te makariri o te vaka* 'the cold of the ship' (*makariri* can be used to mean being cold as well as having a cold, as in the English usage). One woman told me that it was only the mission ship that caused colds and that the government ship was good, but her husband said all ships caused colds. Mission ships tended to stay for a day or two, during which time the crew and passengers for other islands would come ashore. The government ships, on the other hand, usually hove to for a matter of hours only, while returning Tikopians who had been away. The more prolonged contact with the mission ship could have caused more colds. Casual observation suggested to me that a fair number of people caught colds after every ship called. Blowing the ship's siren was also still held to be dangerous to the health of the island. The captains of ships that call regularly at the island are aware of this belief and refrain from doing so, but a new ship on a trial run to the eastern outer islands in 1980 did blow its whistle on departure, which gave rise to angry comment.

The epidemics of colds and coughs, because of their frequency, are most often discussed but there are other diseases recognized as introduced ones. Tuberculosis and malaria are the most serious.

In 1980 there were sixteen people in Tikopia being treated for tuberculosis, although there were many others in whom the disease had been arrested. Most of them had at some stage been hospitalized in Honiara, Kirakira, or Santa Cruz until their condition was stable enough for them to return to Tikopia. Some, however, were still regarded as active carriers of the disease. The nurse had told them all not to share cups, spoons, or pipes with other people or to follow the common practice of chewing a wad of betel nut and transferring it to someone else. Some of the tuberculosis sufferers followed these instructions faithfully but uncomprehendingly. Several of them told me they did not know why these restrictions should be put upon them, but as they wanted to get well they would do what the nurse said. This lack of understanding of the intention behind the nurse's orders sometimes led to practices which could have spread infection. One woman, who otherwise carefully followed the directions of the nurse, spat on a plate and wiped the saliva around with the palm of her hand to clean the plate before putting food on it, an action the nurse had not thought to prohibit specifically.

Malaria is endemic to many parts of the Solomons, although it is not so in Tikopia. It has been responsible for the majority of deaths in the Tikopian settlement of Nukukaisi, on the island of San Cristobal. Others who have suffered attacks and survived have returned to Tikopia but, although all the vectors necessary for the disease to establish itself on Tikopia are present, it does not appear to have done so. A severe fever with intense pain in the joints lasting for three days is common in Tikopia and has been confused with malaria, but a World Health Organization doctor who was investigating malaria in the Eastern Outer Islands Province in 1980 said that the fever was probably sand-fly fever (personal communication, Dr. H. Marshaal). Aspirin from the clinic reduces the discomfort of the fever.

Some non-Tikopian terminology has been adopted to describe certain ailments. The pidgin word *bakua* is used increasingly to describe all skin complaints, although there are several specific words for different types of skin problems in Tikopian. Another introduced word used in a portmanteau fashion is the English word "gonorrhoea," which is applied to any venereal complaint. According to the nurse, one or two men who have been away from the island suffer from it, their infection having been diagnosed in Honiara. There are no laboratory facilities easily available to the nurse in Tikopia for making such tests. During my stay on the island five women came to ask me to treat them for what they said was gonorrhoea. A prohibition on a woman's discussing anything of a sexual nature with men generally, and especially men in certain kin relationships, prevented these women from mentioning their problems to the male nurse. In some cases their symptoms sounded to me like cystitis (frequent urination accompanied by a burning sensation) but I lacked both the knowledge and the medication to be of any help, and although I went to the nurse on their behalf he seemed reluctant to bring the matter up with the women concerned.

Both new disease and new remedies have been introduced to Tikopia. Tikopians who have worked in other parts of the Solomons have brought back patent medicines such as cough mixtures, preparations against headlice and ringworm, and a very popular nostrum from Taiwan called "White Flower," which smells strongly of camphor and is advertised as a preventative against cholera and typhoid. This potion is used for colds, sores, and headaches, taken internally or applied externally.

After the Second World War a dresser was sent to Tikopia by the Solomon Islands government. The dresser was a paramedical practitioner, equipped with a small supply of medications such as antimalarials, antifungicides, and penicillin. His job was to treat minor complaints, leaving more serious ones for the occasional medical patrols. In the 1950s and 1960s some Tikopians, both male and female, trained as nurses at the Honiara hospital and were assigned to positions around the Solomons, but not to Tikopia where there were no facilities for them. The Tikopians had applied to the provincial government for funds to construct a clinic and pay a nurse, but their request was ignored and finally in the 1970s they built a clinic themselves with money from the Tikopia Development Fund on the understanding that the province would pay the nurse's salary. The nurse in 1980 was a male Tikopian.

By 1980 the clinic had become very dilapidated. The kerosene refrigerator no longer worked. Until the end of 1980, no ship calling at the island had the refrigeration facilities to transport medicines taken from cold store at Santa Cruz hospital, two or three days away by ship. There are two rooms in which seriously ill people can sleep at the Tikopia clinic and the nurse is able to receive directions from the doctor at Santa Cruz by radiotelephone during Tikopia's one hour of transmission time each day. The provincial government will pay the fare of anyone who needs to be sent to hospital for urgent treatment but not for matters like investigation of the cause of sterility. There are no facilities for X-rays, the setting of broken bones, extraction of teeth, or any type of laboratory testing. In 1980 there was no thermometer on the island.

The treatments and remedies available from the clinic include weight and blood pressure checks on pregnant women, treatments for fevers and skin diseases, Depo-Provera contraceptive injections which about twenty women receive, and tuberculosis treatment. Babies are born at home but the nurse sends a sterile razor for cutting the cord and has drugs for postpartum bleeding or retained placenta. The consulting room has an uncurtained wire mesh window and people waiting to see the nurse watch and listen to the activity inside the surgery. This exposure precludes some types of physical examination and deters questions on matters such as sterility.

Each Tikopian has a group of relatives to whom he or she must show respect. Joking with them is avoided and so is any mention of sexual matters. The Tikopian nurse feels he cannot, for example, speak to village groups about family planning because in each village there are a few people who fall into this category vis-à-vis the nurse. To have a non-Tikopian nurse would eliminate this problem but raise another, that of language. The lingua franca of the Solomons is pidgin English, which most of the women of Tikopia do not speak. The Tikopians themselves would like to have two nurses on the island, a male and a female, but the size of the population does not entitle them to two salaries from the provincial government. They have discussed paying the second salary themselves but there is no source of income on the island, where the life-style is purely subsistence; it could only be done if Tikopians working elsewhere in the Solomons agreed to be levied.

Once or twice a year the doctor from Santa Cruz comes to Tikopia staying for about eight hours each time, and seeing cases the nurse considers serious. Occasionally, specialist teams come to the island to look for malaria or examine eyes. They can only stay for one day and the pressure on their time has caused some unfortunate incidents in the past. A malaria specialist, wishing to check the population for enlarged spleens, asked the nurse to collect the people into large groups and make them lie on the ground. To people who regard the head, especially of men, as sacred, assuming a prone position in public was completely repugnant and the Tikopians refused to cooperate.

It is not only European disease and medicine that contact with the outside world has introduced to Tikopia. They now find themselves living and working with their Melanesian neighbors. This subject will be dealt with in the next section because all the reports I have collected concerning Melanesian influence on Tikopian beliefs deal with magic and sorcery.

Fakafuaa 'Bringing Sickness by Spirit Means'

The assignment of a cause, rather than the recognition of symptoms, is the unifying factor in this category. In some of the instances which will be described, initial diagnosis had been made in terms of symptoms, but when the complaint did not respond to the usual remedy the case was rediagnosed. The general term *fakafuaa* heads this section to suggest that, in western terms, there is a supernatural or spiritual component involved in the illnesses described. The term is quite inadequate to convey the complexity of Tikopian spiritual beliefs, both traditional and Christian, but the case studies will, to a small degree, illustrate the range of diagnoses and remedies used. They are based on several areas of Tikopian belief: belief in a soul; belief in negative powers, either random or harnessed, indigenous or introduced, which could be used to cause sickness or death; and the idea, discussed earlier, that disturbance of the natural or social order is deleterious to the health of the body politic or the body physical.[4]

Tikopians believe that each living human has a soul. *Ora* and *mauri* are terms often used interchangeably to mean "soul," although the Tikopian priest suggested that *mauri* should be used for the soul while it is still in the body, and *ora* for the released soul after death. The soul after death is cleansed of mortality and enters a heaven (Christian and traditional beliefs overlap here) where it becomes an *atua* 'spirit', but if a semblance of the dead person is later seen it is called an *ata* 'ghost'.

It appears that the soul of a living person is partially detachable. If someone sneezes, bystanders will say "Ora!", which means "life" as well as "soul." This is to call the soul back in case it has been dislodged by the sneeze, and it is especially said to young children whose souls are less firmly attached. It is also believed that the soul travels during sleep, its activities being the sleeper's dreams. The appearance of one person in the dreams of another can be regarded as a meeting between their souls, but sometimes it is believed that a nonhuman spirit can take the appearance of a living person in the dreams of another, intending to deceive or frighten. I was given no consistent explanation of the way in which a dreamer could distinguish between the two manifestations except by discussing the dreams which seemed significant with others. It was thought that dreams, sometimes in a straightforward manner or at other times couched symbolically, could contain information about death or sickness as well as matters like fishing conditions.

It seemed to me, although my informants did not make it explicit, that there is an element of ubiquity about the soul which allows it to maintain the life of its possessor while traveling in dreams or traveling in reality (a case below illustrates this latter point). It was also apparent that the soul, especially when in a dispersed condition, is vulnerable to loss or attack.

The idea that malevolence, especially arising out of the displeasure of the powerful, can cause epidemics and other disasters has already been mentioned with reference to a bishop and the ships of the Melanesian Mission. Traditionally, there is a precedent for this belief. The Atua Lasi, premier god of the Tikopian pantheon, is controller of disease. When a group of people under his protection were killed, in revenge he released an epidemic on the land and scores more died (Firth 1967, 288). The *ariki* of Tikopia are still believed to have the power to *tautuku* 'curse' someone causing their illness or death. But it is not only powerful gods and humans who can cause sickness. Ill health and misfortune can be caused variously by offended relatives, both living and dead; by *atua vare* 'malicious spirits', who, having been neither god nor human, resemble European elementals, spirits of earth and trees and the shore; and by sorcery from other islands. The system of belief in spirit-caused sickness is self-validating, as will be seen. It is also internally consistent and sufficiently flexible to incorporate both Christianity and western medicine. Traditionally,

> Simple ailments and injuries were treated by the Tikopia as chance occurrences, curing themselves. . . . The attribution of spirit causation was left fairly open. But in any persistent illness, or grave sudden illness, diagnosis was usually sought from a spirit medium. (Firth 1970, 274)

After his third visit to Tikopia in 1966, Firth reported that spirit mediumship had ceased; the demand for the therapeutic service it offered had been diminished by the development of local medical facilities. In its place, prayer and the laying on of hands by the Christian priest catered to the more psychological needs of the sick (Firth 1970, 295–96).

By 1980, despite church and clinic, there was again reference to the spirit component in the diagnosis of sickness, and a few spirit mediums had returned to their traditional practice. The spirit medium or *vaka atua*, literally "vessel of the spirit," was possessed by a spirit which, speaking through the mouth of the medium, diagnosed illness and predicted its resolution. Spirit possession could be induced by the medium or might come upon the *vaka atua* without his or her conscious volition. Male mediums appeared to be more in control of the possessing spirits, female mediums more at their mercy. The possessing spirits were sometimes ancestral spirits, but there were others who had never been human.

The following case studies illustrate some of these points.

Case study 1. This example deals with the dangers of social disharmony to the health of a young child whose soul was not yet firmly attached to his body. The child was suffering from diarrhoea and was becoming very listless and dehydrated, so he was taken to the clinic and given some medicine by the nurse. When there was no immediate improvement a neighbor pointed out that the parents had been quarrelling a lot and that it was unlikely the baby would recover until harmony was restored to the household. The church has introduced the idea of confession of sin and, especially before Easter and Christmas, the congregation is exhorted to confess bad feelings and bad behavior to one another or to the priest so that social equilibrium can be restored. Ill health or infertility can be caused by domestic disharmony, as poor crops can be caused by wider social disharmony. In this case, the parents admitted their quarrelling to the priest, who blessed them, and their baby recovered.

Case study 2. This case is about social disturbances and their effect on a soul divided. A Tikopian man visiting Honiara fell sick and his body became cold and deathlike. Another Tikopian gave the sick man a decoction of leaves of the *varovaro (Premna corymbosa)* to drink and he soon recovered. Later it was discovered that on the day the man in Honiara fell ill, other men in Tikopia had been fighting drunkenly in his house in Tikopia, disturbing that part of his soul which had remained at home and causing his body to fall ill in Honiara. While diagnosis of the cause was not made at the time of the treatment, the sick man's symptoms seemed so severe to his companion that the medicine was administered with an invocation to a powerful clan god.

Case study 3. This case deals with an illness which has not yet happened. A woman was unkind to her elderly and ailing father-in-law with whom she and her husband lived. She spoke harshly to the older man and offered him very little food, accusing him of bringing sickness into the house which might harm her children and of taking food from their mouths. This was truly shocking behavior on her part in a society where a daughter-in-law must show extreme respect to her father-in-law and, although her husband and the priest remonstrated with her, she persisted. Finally the father-in-law lay on his sleeping mat and refused to take any food. People related to him on his mother's side brought him food and begged him to eat, but he refused and soon died. The nurse told me that the old man had cirrhosis of the liver from many years of hard drinking in Honiara and that he had been sent home to die, but popular opinion in his village was that his daughter-in-law had shamed him and caused him to die.

Social disapproval had failed to change the woman's behavior and I expressed surprise to a friend that her husband had not taken stronger action, as indeed a Tikopian husband was entitled to do. My friend said that the woman was headstrong and difficult to control but that her punishment would inevitably come—either she or one of her children would get sick and die because her father-in-law would curse her from the spirit world. Obviously, in this case, the first serious sickness to strike the household would be seen as the old man's retribution. Such stories of punishment from the spirit world for dereliction of duty were legion.

Case study 4. A person who has not obviously offended against his fellow men may also be stricken with a serious sickness, and this event can be encompassed by a belief in malevolent spirits which are not ancestral ones.

A man became very ill with a high fever, and as treatment at the clinic did not help him, a spirit medium was consulted. The medium went into a trance and was told by his possessing spirit that the sick man had gone to the lake to bathe, always at the same spot, where a female spirit, lusting after him, had taken advantage of his regular appearance to have sexual intercourse with him, although he was not aware of it. In the spirit world she had borne him a son and a daughter. Now, to complete her family, she wanted him to die so he could come live with them.

Once the medium had discovered the cause of the man's sickness he was able to call on a powerful clan spirit who had a detachable man-eating tooth. The tooth was sent to kill the two spirit children and, this accomplished, the man recovered. Similar cases of spirit intercourse causing sickness in both men and women were reported.

Case study 5. There was a strong tendency in Tikopia for sick people to try several different remedies at once. A man came to my house with what appeared to be an abscessed tooth—his cheek was swollen and he was in great pain. The nurse had no facilities for pulling teeth and he had given the sufferer painkillers which were not controlling the pain for long. I had some antibiotics and I went to his village each day for seven days to administer one. After a week the swelling and pain had gone. I asked the man what treatments he had had besides those of the nurse and my antibiotics. He said his mother had told him to chew a certain leaf, and that his cousin who had a bottle of holy oil (coconut oil blessed by a priest) had drawn a cross on his sore cheek. When I asked which of the remedies had worked, he said it had been the holy oil. Apparently, he had been working alone in his garden when night fell and this had made him vulnerable to attack by malevolent bush spirits. His sore face started the next day, confirming his fear that he had indeed been attacked, but the holy oil had finally countered it.

Case study 6. A woman, married for two years, had not been able to conceive a child. The nurse was unable to help and could only recommend that the couple go to a hospital on another island for tests. This couple could not afford the fare and their strategies first to conceive and then to carry and bear the child successfully were many.

They asked the priest to pray for them, and the chief of their clan, in whose hands was the power to heal and bless, to touch the woman.

Finally she conceived, but during her pregnancy she was unwell and was also troubled by uneasy dreams about the death of the child and herself. She told her dreams to her uncle, a practicing spirit medium, and he divined that leaf magic from the New Hebrides was being used against her. A leaf buried beside one of the house posts would cause her to lose the baby and die herself. The reason for this foreign sorcery was that a branch of her husband's family, into which a New Hebridean had married two generations previously, stood to gain valuable garden lands if she did not produce a son, and apparently it was this group that had taken steps to bring her death about. The pregnant woman countered the leaf sorcery by moving to another house for the rest of her pregnancy, asking a group of Franciscan brothers who were visiting the island to pray for her and, through the offices of her spirit-medium uncle, requesting the protection of clan spirits. The successful delivery of her son was attributed to the Franciscans.[5]

Case study 7. Many forms of mental disturbance are recognized in Tikopia, such as simple-mindedness, periodic insanity, passing spells of odd behavior, and so on. Spirit intervention is believed to be responsible in most cases, although it was also said that madness tends to run in certain families for no known reason. (Albinism was also seen as a hereditary trait, but it was usually thought to have been introduced by men from other islands who had married Tikopian women.)

This example deals with the power of curses, both Tikopian and Melanesian, to damage both the mind and the body of the person cursed. The youngest son of an *ariki,* a highly intelligent young man, went to Honiara where he trained as a hospital laboratory technician and passed his exams with distinction. He formed a liaison with a Melanesian girl but, bowing to pressure from his family, severed his relationship with her. It was said that her brothers made spells to punish the young Tikopian.

Then, his father, the *ariki,* came to the hospital in Honiara to be treated for tuberculosis. From the time of his accession to the position a Tikopian chief does not cut his hair. The welfare of the land resides in, and is symbolized by, the body of the chief, and if he cuts his hair it is believed that he will be cutting off the lives of some of his people. The son, embarrassed by his father's long hair in the modern hospital, begged the old man to cut it. The shocked *ariki* cursed him for his unfilial (and un-Tikopian) behavior.

The son returned to Tikopia, where his mind and body deteriorated. The two curses *(tautuku)* had been put on him some five years before my arrival on the island. By 1980 he was emaciated, filthy, and mute. He rarely ate unless ordered to do so by his eldest brother and his behavior was irrational. It was generally believed that both curses were responsible for his changed condition, the curse of a chief and a father being very strong but the curse from another island being very dangerous.

Case study 8. This final and more complex case study, which deals with the family of the resident priest, reflects the interplay of the many factors affecting attitudes to sickness and healing in Tikopia.

Nau M, the wife of the priest, had been unwell and was returning from a visit to the clinic when Nau F, an old woman who was a spirit medium and mother of a chief, called to her. The old lady said that a spirit had told her that Nau M would die of her sickness, which had been caused by the anger of the priest's late grandfather, Pu M. This man, who died in the Russell Islands a few years before, had himself been a well known spirit medium before his conversion to Christianity. Nau M, understandably upset, told her husband of her encounter and he went to see Nau F, demanding that she call her possessing spirit so that he could talk to it. The spirit returned and repeated through the medium that Nau M would die because Pu M was angry that his funeral rites had not been adequately conducted. The priest then asked the spirit how it knew that his wife was sick and it replied that it could see inside her body. Father M said that only doctors who had studied such things could see inside the body and that Tikopians were ignorant of its workings; futhermore, the island now believed in God, who was more powerful than the old spirits. The spirit replied that he had seen God, who was like a burning fire. Father M then told the spirit to go away, threatening to exorcise it if it returned, and he warned Nau F to stop calling the spirit as "it made the faith of the half-Christian waver."

Nau F did not become possessed again for a month or so. I heard people saying that the breadfruit crop would fail because the spirits of her clan were responsible for the strong growth of the breadfruit, and if Nau F was forbidden to talk to them they would abandon their responsibilities.

Some two months after the priest's warning to the old medium, his father became very ill. The nurse treated him, prayers were said in church for his recovery, and two of the *ariki* came to lay hands on him. Then, one day the priest's mother passed Nau F, who said, "Tomorrow you will cry." Her possessing spirit had told her that the man would die the next day, and again Pu M, grandfather of the priest and father of the ill man, was blamed. The death occurred as she foretold.

This was a time of great trial for the priest. One of his sisters had a child of about eighteen months who became extremely ill at the time the priest's father was sick, and the two patients were moved into Father M's house. I had heard that the child, who was suffering from diarrhoea, had been fed some very hot food by a careless young aunt and it had burned his mouth so badly he was refusing to eat anything at all. The combination of diarrhoea and the lack or nourishment was causing the child to deteriorate rapidly. In this situation everyone intervened. Father M prayed for the child and insisted he be given cool, boiled water only, as that was what Europeans did in Honiara. The nurse gave the child an injection of penicillin. I tried to get him to drink milk powder mixed with boiled water, into which I had put a crushed anti-diarrhoea tablet. Another medium (not Nau F) called on the spirits, who said the illness was being caused by the late Pu M. Finally the infant's mother managed to get him to take some watery mashed pumpkin and he started to improve, his improvement being attributed to the spirit medium's intervention.

Then a further disaster hit the family. Father M's other sister had an adopted child of about four years of age. The real father of this child was a Melanesian mission priest who was, at that time, assigned to a parish elsewhere in the Solomons. On a Thursday evening, the priest and his brother-in-law (the adoptive father) went visiting relatives in another village while their wives, the adopted child, and some teenage girls remained in the priest's house. In the early hours of the morning someone appeared at the door, saying to one of the girls that she must go to call the priest and his brother-in-law. The girl said that she recognized the figure at the door as the dead grandmother of the adopted child. By the time someone fetched the two men, the child was found to be lying cold and apparently lifeless. The priest prayed over the child, and by daylight on Friday he had recovered. Later that day the nurse was called and he gave the child an injection, whereupon the boy went into convulsions. Through Friday night the priest nursed the child and prayed for him, and by Saturday morning he seemed better. Sometime during that day a young man, also related to the child, administered a few drops of White Flower (the camphor-smelling potion mentioned earlier). Soon afterwards the nurse returned, gave the child another injection, and he died almost immediately.

This case illustrates very clearly the mélange of responses to illness: prayer and the nurse's injections, ancestral spirits who both curse and warn, and a patent medicine. But the apportioning of blame was interesting. The concensus of opinion in the village was that Pu M's angry spirit was responsible. The appearance of the dead grandmother was seen as a beneficent intervention on behalf of the child. The priest denied this and said that his grandfather had been given an appropriate burial, that his own father's death had been brought about by his intemperate habits, and that the death of the adopted child was the fault of the nurse who should not have given the second injection after the first one caused convulsions.

The interrelationship between Christianity and traditional beliefs and practices is an interesting one. When lay people resorted to a mixture of remedies it was usually the power of prayer or the efficacy of holy oil that was credited with the successful resolution of a health problem. In the case of the misfortunes which affected the priest's family, both the cause of the illnesses and deaths and the cure of one of those involved were attributed to ancestral spirits.

CONCLUSION

Although much of the Pacific was converted to Christianity one hundred fifty years ago and, with increasing contact, has been for many years exposed to western medicines and ideas about health, Tikopia's experience has been quite different. The small size and isolation of the island protected it from the depredations of those who were exploiting land and people elsewhere in the Pacific. A century ago other small islands, their populations reduced by introduced epidemic disease and blackbirders, lost their older people, the leaders and repositories of traditional knowledge. Tikopia retained its traditional religious practices well into the twentieth century, and it was only after the loss of significant pagan leaders during an influenza epidemic in the 1950s that the island became entirely Christian. The introduction of western medicine has also occurred largely since the Second World War and is still at a very simple level, administered by a nurse. The late introduction of both western religion and medicine meant that it occurred at a time when the attitudes of missionaries and medical educators were more liberal toward traditional practices. Tikopia's first resident priest, a man from the Banks Islands, married a Tikopian woman, learned the language, and, in his fifty years on the island, came to an understanding of the people. After his death another Melanesian priest was assigned to Tikopia for three years, during which time he rigorously tried to extirpate all manifestations of traditional customs including healing practices. This brief period was the only time in which the culture of Tikopia came under serious attack and since then the priests have been local men. In their teaching of Christianity they naturally disapprove of any rituals, such as spirit mediumship, having to do with the gods and spirits of the pagan religion. However, while a foreign priest might say that the traditional spirits do not exist, the Tikopian priests forbid communication with them, thereby tacitly admitting their existence. Equally, medical training organizations, cultural publications, and radio programs throughout the Solomons have been increasingly encouraging the collection and dissemination of information about traditional healing practices, some of which are seen as complementary to introduced health services. Thus, historical and geographical factors have combined to preserve much of Tikopian tradition, including ideas about sickness and healing.

The traditional Tikopian view of sickness held that there were minor complaints for which herbal remedies were efficacious, and there were serious or sudden afflictions whose onset was due to a negative power emanating from either human or supernatural sources. The sufferer was in some cases believed to have attracted illness by offending, wittingly or unwittingly, against a person or an ideal of behavior. In other cases the illness was thought to be caused by the motiveless malevolence of someone or something powerful. The dual explanation of serious illness, as a punishment or as the result of malice, provided an extremely flexible model which both reinforced the island's social order and accommodated the intrusion of elements from outside. This scheme was reiterated in both concrete and metaphorical terms.

It is possible to stand on the highest part of Tikopia, the peak of the sacred mountain Reani, and see the whole island, a small piece of land in an ocean which stretches empty to the horizon in every direction. From their travels the Tikopians know that other lands exist many days' sailing away, but, apart from their nearest neighbor Anuta, these are places where the language and customs differ greatly from those of Tikopia and where the people, in the past, may have been contacted only in aggression. It is therefore easy to understand the Tikopian idea of the integrity of their island, a bounded entity to be defended from external attack or internal dissension. By quite explicit metaphorical extension the island, as a body of land, is compared with the body politic and the body physical. Threats to the well-being of the body can come from inside the island or from outside. In the case of the land itself, the chiefs had traditionally exhorted the people each year to care for their land and use it sensibly, not overtaxing its resources. Despite their best endeavors, however, a devastating cyclone could wreak havoc, and increasing contact with other islands has recently shown that the land can also be threatened by introduced plant diseases. The political and social well-being of the island is believed to depend on harmonious relationships among the people, combined with the repulsion, if possible, of disruptive external elements. The physical body is believed to reflect these concerns. Internal social disorder can be manifested in physical disease, while external factors, some as apparently motiveless as a cyclone, can effect the body through intervention from the spirit world, from introduced disease, or from foreign magic.

In the treatment of simple ailments such as skin or stomach complaints, the ones the Tikopians refer to as "just sickness," western medicine is thought to be quite effective although traditional remedies are still used, the choice of treatment often being influenced by such factors as distance from the clinic. In the case of more serious illnesses, Tikopian beliefs about possible causes are fairly clear, but the assignment of cause and prescription of remedy in any specific case are less so. Both diagnosis and treatment of a complaint can be, and often are, simultaneously carried out by a priest, nurse, spirit medium, or local herbalist. To which of these agencies the cure is attributed is a matter of choice, but it appears that spiritual remedies, either Christian or pagan, are most often given the credit.

NOTES

1. For his reports on pre-Christian ideas about sickness and healing in Tikopia, see, for example, Firth 1967, chaps. 7, 14; 1970, chap. 9 et seq.
2. A description of earlier migrations by Tikopians, their high death rate, and, eventually, more successful schemes for allowing them to live in other parts of the Solomons can be found in Spillius 1957.
3. All plant identifications and many of the glosses used in the translation of Tikopian terms have been taken from works by Raymond Firth.
4. For detailed descriptions of Tikopian beliefs about the soul, and the practice of spirit mediumship, see especially Firth 1967, chaps. 14, 15; and Firth 1970.
5. The attribution of efficacy to one form of treatment rather than another has its dangers. A man who desperately wanted a son asked both the priest for his prayers and an elderly relative for a *tama feao* 'fertility magic'. While his wife was still pregnant the man dreamed she was bearing a son and credited it to the church. The spirits invoked by the *tama feao* were so angry that their contribution was not acknowledged that they changed the child (still unborn) into a girl. The woman telling the story said that the priest changed it back again, and all through the woman's pregnancy there was the baby, first a boy and then a girl. Again, the power of the church was believed to have prevailed and the baby was born a boy.

5

Tongan Healing Practices
Claire D. F. Parsons

The Kingdom of Tonga consists of approximately 150 islands, of which about 40 are inhabited. They are scattered in the tropical Pacific between 15 and 22 degrees south of the equator. The islands of the easterly coral belt stretch 750 km and contain the main island groups of Vava'u and Ha'apai as well as Tongatapu and 'Eua in the south. These islands support most of Tonga's population of ninety-five thousand. The people enjoy an unhurried existence founded on a subsistence life-style; they grow staple crops on bush allotments, raise a few pigs and chickens, and fish. The women also weave mats and beat tapa cloth, of which a small amount will be sold along with other handcrafts to the occasional tourist. In the downtown market in Nuku'alofa, Tonga's capital, a limited range of vegetables is available and occasionally bottles of herbal preparations are sold as a general cure-all medicine.

In 1979 I visited Tonga as a sociologist interested in understanding how the Tongan people talk about sickness, what they know and believe about sickness, and what actions they take when sickness enters their lives. To develop this understanding it was necessary to record Tongan views of western healing practices in relation to their own, and also something of the views of the western-trained health personnel in Tonga.[1] I spent seven months in the islands of Kapa and Vava'u, Lifuka in Ha'apai, Tongatapu, and 'Eua. My interviews were initially conducted in English, or with the aid of a Tongan translator, but after several months I had gained sufficient fluency to conduct interviews in Tongan while occasionally referring to another translator to check my understanding. Most of the information presented here was gathered during the last three months of my stay.

AN UNEASY ALLIANCE BETWEEN MEDICAL SYSTEMS

In general, the Tongan public and Health Department officials seem to be at variance over evaluations of the effectiveness of indigenous healing

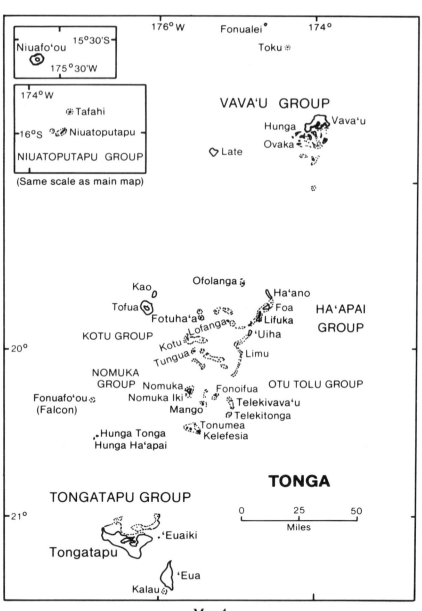

Map 4

practices. Both lay and professional members of Tongan society reported to me that for more than a decade, traditional healing practices have been proscribed by western-trained doctors. Several members reported that it was unlawful to practice traditional healing techniques and that such practitioners could face prosecution. As in other parts of the Pacific, such statements reflect publicized Department of Health policy rather than actual legislative or court practice. While such policies may have some inhibitory effect, they do not result in subterfuge or clandestine performance of traditional medical practice. Over the last decade radio broadcasts have presented western health practices as being the "correct" therapeutic procedure and have challenged overtly, and by implication, the effectiveness of traditional healing methods. It is perhaps not surprising that some Tongans state that they would not always report having tried traditional medicines before seeking treatment for a particular sickness from a hospital doctor. Interestingly, over the last two years radio broadcasts have presented formal debates and discussions between exponents of both modes of healing practice.

Discussions with a number of Tongan Medical Officers (western trained) raised emotive opinions about the effectiveness of traditional healing practices. The variety of accounts seemed to me to be largely influenced by the extent to which the medical officers assumed that I supported western practices, as well as other factors such as an awareness of Health Department policy, the influence of their own specialized training, their practice being situated in a hospital (not in the village among the people), and so forth. There has, however, been recent acknowledgement by the Department's members that traditional methods do have some contribution to make to sickness management. This has coincided with, and is perhaps not unrelated to, similar evaluations presented over the last five years by such international organizations as the World Health Organization (see Preface). The descriptions in the following pages are selected vignettes from the Tongan people who participated in this study and do not necessarily reflect the views of all Tongans.

CONCEPTS OF HEALTH AND SICKNESS

The concept of "health" has been variously defined in the literature of medical science and medical social science, and western notions of health have been demonstrated to be of little or no relevance to the peoples of many nonwestern societies. Health as normality (that which is routinely expected) varies considerably from culture to culture.[2] It is a social construct which has meaning only in the interaction of a particular social group.

In contemporary Tongan society, the term used to convey the concept of health is *mo'ui lelei,* and it has no meaning for the people beyond its introduced meaning. The notion of managing one's daily activities in order to improve and maintain maximum physical health is regarded as western. In Tonga, a healthy life is the maintenance of harmony in relationships among family and community members, both living and deceased (Parsons 1981c).

While the western notion of health may not be relevant in the everyday lives of the Tongan people, the events of sickness are. In Tongan society the term *puke* means to feel physically ill and usually implies nausea (while *lue* means to vomit). The term *mahaki* refers to all forms of sickness, mental, physical, with or without a disease state (pathology) being present. *Mahaki* translates as "disease" or "sickness," which are used interchangeably. Primarily, the category *mahaki* can be reclassified as either a Tongan sickness *(mahaki faka-Tonga)* or a European sickness *(mahaki faka-Pālangi)*. As my discussions with the Tongan people developed it seemed that four general types of Tongan sickness could be identified: *āvanga, fasi, hangatāmaki,* or simply *mahaki,* which is not regarded as belonging to the first three classes. For example, one woman explained to me, "She has what you call a 'stroke,' but we know it as a *mahaki,* not a *hangatāmaki* just as a *mahaki.*"

Āvanga refers to what some researchers have called "spirit sickness" (including spirit possession). The *āvanga,* usually the spirits of recently deceased kin, are occasionally thought to be the indirect agents causing all sickness. Today, however, most Tongans accept the idea of accidental causes and natural causes of sickness as well as supernatural. *Fasi* refers to disorders of the bones and muscles. *Hangatāmaki* refers to disorders of the skin and internal organs. Eye, ear, nose and throat, central nervous system, and many cardiovascular conditions are usually described as being simply *mahaki.*

Deformities and other congenital defects are not considered part of the *mahaki* classification and are usually attributed to the mother's having profaned a *tapu* or misbehaved in some way while she was pregnant.[3] Another condition not interpreted as sickness unless it is severe, is diarrhoea in children, as it is regarded as a normal condition of infants and children.

The term *faito'o* refers to medicine as a cure or therapy. It is also the term used for the healer, and again, as the verb meaning "to heal." The term "patient" is sometimes used but is not translated into Tongan. The Tongans do not have a term that labels and alters the status or role of the sick person as the western term does.

As these examples suggest, concepts of health and sickness are social constructs, relevant to and part of everyday life. To understand this idea further, we turn now to a closer examination of the two primary categories used by Tongans to classify sickness.

WESTERN AND TONGAN SICKNESS

This dual classification assigns certain sicknesses thought to have been introduced by Europeans, or to be most effectively cured by European medicine, to the category *mahaki faka-Pālangi* (Parsons 1981a, 69–83). The remaining sicknesses are assigned to the category *mahaki faka-Tonga*. It is important to this classification that European therapies are considered not only unsuited to treating Tongan sicknesses but also dangerous. Tongan sicknesses require treatment by a *faito'o* or Tongan doctor, and Pālangi sicknesses require treatment by a *toketā* or western healer.

On one occasion, when I asked what would happen if a person sick with *āvanga* were taken to the hospital, I was told: "The hospital cannot do anything. The disease which we call *āvanga* cannot be treated by the doctor. If you take this one to the hospital and he is given an injection, that would be the end [death]. Sometimes he may be operated on, but this would not cure it." The belief that death could result from injections (*huhu*) or tablets (*fo'i'akau*) being given to a Tongan suffering from a Tongan sickness was reiterated many times during my interviews (Parsons 1981a, 70). Some Tongan sicknesses named were *filimamangu, makehekehe, mofi faka-Tonga, mea, ngalo'afu, mata'ika, kulokula, haukiva'e, kahi, pala, mata fa, mavae'ua,* and other diagnostic labels for which there is often no western equivalent.

Although individual accounts can vary over how a particular sickness is to be identified, Tongans do express certainty as to what constitutes a sickness type. The following conversation between two Tongan villagers is an example:

- A. If it's a fever, this is what is difficult. How can mothers tell which kind of fever it is, the *mofi faka-Tonga* or the *mofi faka-Pālangi*?
- B. Listen, I'll tell you. There is a time when our children get a fever. If the fever covers all over the body—up to the feet—it is a *mofi-Pālangi*. If the mother can only feel the fever in the forehead and stomach, and cold elsewhere, then she knows the child must be teething or something. Then she gets the tops of the *hehea* leaves and another kind. When they're applied the baby is cured.
- A. It must be an exact symptom [*faka'ilonga*].
- B. Yes, it's a sure way.
- A. When she's hot all over.
- B. When she's hot all over, they say it's a *mofi-Pālangi*. That's its name, *mofi-Pālangi*. If it isn't the *mofi-Pālangi*, it's the other one. The child may have a temperature and be active but doesn't lose interest in food. The appetite is alright.

A. So there's fever and the child is active, and another one where the child appears very, very weak.

The certainty expressed is an important feature of the process of problem identification. People must "know" how to act. Therefore, although the classification of two basic sickness types fixes, or makes factual, what is essentially a fluctuating phenomenon, it is most important to Tongans that this classification be the first step in the diagnosis of illness.

The importance placed on the ability to diagnose a Tongan or European sickness is reflected in a statement made by an 'Eua woman while we were in an open shed stacking baskets, which had been woven for sale in New Zealand. The villager commented, "I spoke to the woman the other day about the baby who died recently. Some said he suffered from measles, some said it was a *mahaki faka-Tonga*. I believe the greatest disadvantage was that the mother was unable to choose which was which." A number of the other women present agreed with the woman's comment. It is part of everyday thinking that error in this first diagnostic step (problem identification) can have, literally, fatal consequences.

Common sicknesses assigned to the Pālangi category include typhoid, influenza, measles, chickenpox, encephalitis, venereal diseases, dengue fever, and respiratory conditions such as tuberculosis, asthma, and pneumonia. Tongans do not assign only the "minor" illnesses to the category *mahaki faka-Tonga*. They have traditionally dealt with fractures of the bones and internal conditions ranging from gynecological disorders to cardiac and respiratory ones.

Reclassification of illnesses can occur when it appears that European medicine will provide a more effective treatment, but it is made more difficult when the alternate therapies do not bring expected results. A public health nurse commented,

> The same thing happens when they come to the hospital. They bring someone over for fever. We give injections and they don't work. So they turn to Tongan medicine and he is cured. Then there's those who try all sorts of cures—say for fever, thinking it's *pala*—and yet when they're taken to the hospital, they're cured. Likewise with fever that covers all over the body: they're taken to the hospital and given injections for three or four days, and it doesn't work. So they introduce Tongan medicine, which clears it.

Since most Tongans expect that therapies that are going to be effective will be so in three to four days, it is perhaps not surprising that western therapies, seldom effective within this period of time, are not generally felt to be an improvement over traditional therapies.

The sicknesses which have most readily been reassigned to the Pālangi category are those which are thought to require surgery, especially when there is acute abdominal pain, such as in appendicitis, hernias, or perforated ulcers. On the whole, though, Tongans see hospitals and clinics as negative if necessary places, and surgery is feared as a portent of death. It is widely believed that the probability of death during or following surgery will be greater than the probability of recovery.

Pālangi therapies are sought according to two implicit rules: (1) the sickness must be of the Pālangi type, or (2) the sickness must be so life threatening that as a second resort one will try anything. In acute, severe conditions, especially with serious pain such as appendicitis, ruptures, burns, hemorrhages, and multiple visible traumas, the *toketā* may even become the first resort for therapy.

To complicate matters further, while differentiating between classes of sickness Tongans also regard certain sicknesses within each class as being treatable by either a western or a Tongan healer. While this might seem to contradict the widespread belief that death can ensue from inappropriate therapy, it is within the flexibility of Tongan reasoning to see that some sicknesses, while being classed as *mahaki faka-Tonga,* can also be interpreted as suited to treatment by either a *faito'o* or a *toketā*. The interpretive process is malleable and pragmatic in practice, and the actual criteria for the decision making are negotiated in each situation. Some of the factors that enter into such decisions are the complexity of the symptoms, the views of the family members involved in the decision making, an assessment of the capabilities of the local *faito'o* whose *mahaki* this particular sickness is thought to be, how many *faito'o* have already been consulted, and past experience with the hospital personnel. The sicknesses which are considered to be treatable by either practitioner usually get established as such through "kinship stories" relating a family's experience of the success of the therapies, and through something as simple as propinquity. Living near one of the four hospitals increases the probability that a Pālangi cure will be sought for what might be classified as a Tongan sickness.

These factors make problematic the matter of locating "order of curative resort," that is, where people routinely go when seeking therapies for their sicknesses. This seeking of predictive patterns of human behavior by health professionals is an attempt to concretize what is in practice a flexible and reflexive process.[4]

TONGAN SICKNESS

Within the category of *mahaki faka-Tonga* four subcategories have emerged in Tongan sickness explanation as a means of further organizing sickness experience. The Tongan method of establishing order in the array of sickness troubles they experience has been to construct four classifications: *āvanga, fasi, hangatāmaki,* and *mahaki*. No matter how the sickness trouble was to be classified, it was traditionally believed that the supernatural order, the spirits, both ancestral and recently deceased kinsmen, were the harbingers of such problems afflicting humankind.[5] A prominent member of Tongan society asserts today that

> the principal causative agent of all sickness is the *āvanga* which traditionally requires three agents or vehicles in order to complete the cycle of health, illness and restoration, or death. These three are the *vaka* or vessel which may take the form of a lizard, or shark, or object, or physical element such as the wind, sun or rain, etc. The second is the *taula* or boat anchor which is interpreted as the priest, that is, a human medium. The third element was the *faletapu* or house where the priest conducted his ritual.

Although similar accounts of traditional beliefs and practices have been transmitted to students of Tongan culture through the writings of Gifford (1929) and other early European visitors, these details do not constitute the everyday, common knowledge of most members of Tongan society. Most Tongans, however, are familiar with the concept of the *āvanga* being "responsible" for sickness and premature death, even if they do not all believe in the existence of the *āvanga*. There are, as we shall see, varying interpretations in the ways they speak of the *āvanga* and of the other categories of Tongan sickness. First, we consider the *āvanga* disorders.

Āvanga

Although the Tongans have several names for the souls or spirits of the dead, the term *āvanga* has traditionally been used to identify the spirit's capacity to inflict sickness, misfortune, or death. The term has also been used to identify a particular type of sickness, one where the individual's physical state seems to be unchanged, yet the behavior so deviates from the normal that the person is obviously greatly "disturbed." That is, as there was no physical manifestation, the label *āvanga* was retained not only as the causative label but also as the classificatory label for this sickness type. In these instances the spirits are thought not only to have caused the sickness but also to be manifest within the individual. These *āvanga* are rarely considered to be ancestral spirits and typically are identified as the ghosts or souls of recently deceased members of the community, usually kinsmen of the person who has been "possessed."

The coming of the missionaries brought the word "devil," which became, in Tongan, *tevolo*. The parallel between the malevolent activities of the *āvanga* and those of the *tevolo* was readily apparent, and the new word quickly became applied to the *āvanga,* especially by Europeans. Rather than being equated with the biblical devil, however, the *āvanga* are usually construed by Tongans as belonging to a domain separate from Christianity. Thus the Tongan people choose to deal with such spirits through their own (secular) means, usually by bringing in a *faito'o āvanga* 'spirit healer', particularly in cases of possession. In some parts of Tonga it has been reported that a family member can cure the sickness without recourse to a specialist healer.

Not all spirits "possess" people in the sense of entering the body and controlling behavior. Some may simply wander about, most often at night, and their presence is indicated by unusual noises in the dark, by "sightings" of faces at windows or in dreams, or simply by the evidence of barking dogs. As elsewhere, it is commonly believed in Tonga that animals sense their presence more readily than do humans.

During the daytime spirits may be encountered almost anywhere, but certain areas, such as graveyards, the bush,[6] or out at sea, are regarded as the most dangerous. When approaching, being in, or departing from any of the numerous graveyards scattered throughout the villages and home sections *('api)* in Tonga, care must be taken not to laugh, shout, sing, whistle, play, eat, excrete, or wear flowers. Most Tongans believe that disrespectful behavior around a graveyard will make one vulnerable to "attack" by spirits (Parsons 1981a, 98). Whistling was reported to me as being a *tapu,* as the act of whistling summons up the spirits, or a spirit. Other accounts recorded in the fieldwork reported that whistling is customarily disapproved of but is not a *tapu.* Indeed whistling will only occasionally be heard and the only time I have heard a Tongan whistle was a young man who was walking across his home ground *('api).*

A diagnosis of spirit possession is based on a number of signs and symptoms *(faka'ilonga),* including bizarre talking, irrational anger, attacking family members, running away and hiding, crying out, swearing and hysteria *(āvea),* and greatly increased strength. The victim of spirit possession, however, is never held accountable for his or her behavior while possessed, and there seems to be no stigma attached to the sickness.

In recent years, the management of spirit sickness in countries such as Tonga has been complicated by the advent of western psychiatry. People thought by some to be afflicted by the *āvanga* are vulnerable to the relabeling of the western psychiatrist and thus may be regarded as having a "psychiatric illness" such as schizophrenia, manic depression, or acute psychosis.[7] This relabeling is problematic, to say the least. When it leads to the application of a different therapy, which can include the introduction of drugs, hospitalization, or even incarceration in prison, what was traditionally an acute but readily cured "illness" can become, in many instances, a long-term psychiatric disturbance.

Fasi

For some Tongans, all sickness is caused by spirits; they therefore lack a concept of "accidental" cause. Other Tongans do accept the notion of accidents and of naturally caused illness such as a skin or wound infection, while still maintaining that certain kinds of sickness are the result of the *āvanga*. The *fasi* disorders are perhaps most readily associated with accidents or natural occurrences as this category includes bone fractures *(fasi)*, dislocations *(homo)*, muscular conditions such as sprains of the ankle *(tapeva)*, ruptures, aches, and so on.

The diagnosis of these conditions is based on the signs and symptoms presented or reported by the injured person. In addition to asking "what happened" and how the person "feels," the healer *(faito'o fasi)* palpates the part of the body causing discomfort to determine whether touching markedly increases the pain and whether any deformity that may not be visible can be felt. The type and degree of pain *(langa; langa'o e uoua* 'pain of the muscle', *langa'o e hui* 'pain of the bone') are significant indicators, as are swelling, redness, and bruised or traumatized tissue and blood *(toto)*.

It is worth noting that there is little difference, apart from the use of X-rays, between the diagnostic methods used by Tongan and western healers. Causal accounts and the kind of therapy applied, however, will vary. The *faito'o* I observed and spoke with told me that an X-ray of the affected part was unnecessary, as they had sufficient means available for diagnosis. They can "feel" the broken bone or dislocation, just as they can "feel" a muscular condition which no X-ray will reveal. In any event, there was little discussion of the diagnostic process. The healers simply "knew" which type of disorder it was after having examined the injured person.

Causal explanations by those whose beliefs revolve around the *āvanga* are offered in such statements as "the spirit 'pushed' the victim." But where the disorder is understood to be the result of a natural occurrence, minimal explanation seems to be required. The sickness talk concerning *fasi* disorders is usually limited to locating the signs and symptoms which provide the diagnostic criteria for assigning a particular label to the condition, especially where bone fractures or dislocations are involved. To the Tongans, these conditions seem to be self-evident, and as there is little or no enigma therapy is soon begun.

The *faito'o fasi* are generally well respected among both lay and professional members of the Tongan society, and there is abundant testimony to the success of their methods. In 1965, out of Tonga's population of 73,729, only ten fractures of any kind were treated by western doctors, and this proportion has not increased significantly since then.

Hangatāmaki *and* Mahaki

According to Gifford (1929, 338), the *hangatāmaki* classification refers to "any sickness or disease appearing on the surface of the body." *Hangatāmaki* literally means "boil," but for Tongans the term has come to include all skin lesions, infections, ulcerations, tumors, inflammations, rashes, and so on. Moreover, the term can also be applied to internal disorders such as of the chest or abdomen and also conditions of the scalp, eyes, ears, nose, and throat. Thus in this one category have been gathered a medley of miscellaneous signs and symptoms which are labeled as various sickness types, including ones which have been recently introduced. Many Tongans, however, interpret the newer disorders (and some of the traditional ones, such as those of the scalp, ears, eyes, nose, and throat) as being not of the *hangatāmaki* classification but rather of a fourth type, that is, *mahaki*. Evidently, then, the *hangatāmaki* category is the one which involves the greatest variation in individual accounts, and those who wish to establish a clear line of demarcation between *hangatāmaki* and *mahaki* will seek an elusive goal.

Within the category *hangatāmaki* is a group of semi-ulcerative conditions known as *pala*. This subcategory is further divided into various types (*pala fefie mate, pala fefie sausau, pala fefie momona, pala fefie pakupaku,* etc.), all of which are described as types of *pala* of the mouth or as other internal *pala*. In addition, there are external *pala* which are recognized by the *faito'o* who specializes in treating these conditions. Distinctions are therefore made which correspond to the limits of a particular healer's practice. In the case of *pala* one healer may treat the internal *pala* and another the external ones. When a healer says, "This is my *mahaki*" or "This is not my *mahaki*," he or she is establishing a range of practice. If the diagnosis indicates an unfamiliar condition, or one that the healer does not feel qualified to cure, the person is told that the sickness is not that healer's specialty, and will usually be directed to another healer.

Another condition regarded as a *hangatāmaki* is *mavae'ua*, which is observed in newborn infants. Two western-trained public health nurses told me that they instruct women at village meetings that the condition called *mavae'ua* is the normal aperture of the infant's fontanelles between the occipital and parietal bones and that this "gap" will close naturally and requires no treatment. In spite of this instruction, the *mahaki mavae'ua* continues to be regarded as a sickness, and it is common knowledge that a particularly restless or sleepy baby is so because of the "gap in his head." This condition (restlessness or sleepiness plus the noted aperture between the skull bones) is taken seriously, and Tongans believe that it requires appropriate treatment by a *faito'o*.

Author. What happens if the cure doesn't work? I mean, can it happen that the treatment of the baby doesn't make the baby better?

Healer. Yes, sometimes the crying and restlessness continue. Then they may look for other things [reasons]. Maybe it is the *āvanga*.

Author. What would happen if a baby suffering from *mavae'ua* isn't taken to the *faito'o* for treatment?

Healer. It would die.

This dialogue illustrates a common logic in Tongan sickness talk: when a sickness is particularly severe or persistent and resists what is considered to be the appropriate therapy, then perhaps it is a case of intervention by the spirits. This kind of connection is made more readily with some conditions than others, for example, those with which the *āvanga* have been associated in the past. One villager explained a particular kind of headache called *haukiva'e:*

Woman. It is different from just a headache which comes and goes quickly. Maybe you try *faito'o* [medicine] or massage; maybe you try the aspirin, but the headache, it goes on. This is *haukiva'e*. Then you know it is a *mahaki faka-Tonga*. They [the healer] treat you. You lie on the floor and the corner of the mat is put over the affected side of your head, and the healer steps on the covered head, rocking the foot onto the face [a kind of massage]. Now if you are not better after the treatment, then you know it is the spirit.

Author. What spirit?

Woman. Well, if it is you [a woman], you go to your mother's grave. If you are a man, you go to your father's grave. You take out the skull, because it is your mother trying to tell you, by giving you a headache, that something is wrong. You break the skull and look for a root or something growing or lying in the head. You take the skull and the root or needle; you take them to the sea and throw them away. Then take the bones back to the grave again. Your headache will go then.

Some people reported "smashing the skull"; others reported "poking the stick in to push the thing [offending object] out." Some said the skull should be washed out; others said to throw the skull into the sea. There seemed to be total agreement, however, that if the person with the *haukiva'e* was female, then a female relative, usually the mother or grandmother, needed to be exhumed and treated as above; the reverse applied for a male.[8]

One young man's condition was described as being caused by the *āvanga* because of its persistence, previous treatment having brought no remission. He had experienced a painful abdomen for several months. "We took out his father's body [from the grave] and took out the part of the stomach [abdominal contents] and burnt it. This was so the disease would not come back and go from generation to generation. The trouble will stop now." The account demonstrates a belief that *āvanga*-induced physical illnesses will recur throughout generations if not dealt with effectively. Thus the family would persist in experiencing a *mahaki fakafāmili* and in this case it would be a *lange kete fāmili*.

I did not meet anyone able or willing to discuss details of the origins of Tongan medical knowledge or how these traditional disease names were derived and the classifications made. There was felt to be no relevance in doing so, since all that is required in day-to-day existence is knowledge of diagnostic and therapeutic procedures. Yet it is interesting in this regard to consider the identification of new sickness types and the creation of new therapies. A teacher of Tongan customs remarked to his students,

> *Manatu* is a new sickness. It is a Tongan sickness because the Pālangi cannot cure it. *Manatu* refers to memory; it means to remember or a remembrance. Here it refers to a disease afflicting small children whose parents, either one or both, are overseas. Usually these are parents overstaying in New Zealand. The children have an elevated temperature, loss of appetite, listlessness, and reluctance to play. They are also often sleepy. I treat these children. They come to me from all over Tonga. I treat them with a macerate using the bark of the *liana* vine and use another for flavor. I have one hundred percent success.

This speaker also referred to the condition of *manatu* as "overstayers sickness," and regarded an elevated temperature, among the various diagnostic signs, as particularly important. The cure is called *vai manatu*.

Another newly diagnosed sickness is called *lolo mai*. The sickness reflects certain disturbances of modern living. In other words, there would seem to be a relationship between *lolo mai* and adaptation to changes occurring in traditional modes of relating (Parsons 1984). An account of *lolo mai* as reported by a Fiji-trained medical officer appeared in the local hospital bulletin.

> Since most or all of us do take turns as Out Patients Officers, how many times do we come across people saying that they have these *"lolo mai"* attacks. More often, one is bound to see at least one or more such patients in a week. . . . Most describe it as a FEELING OF GENERALIZED WEAKNESS, some experience it as numbness, others say that it is "death," still others refer to it as a loss of power or energy. Whatever the feeling might be it GRADUALLY

> CRAWLS UPWARDS (FROM THE LOWER LIMBS OR LOWER ABDOMINAL REGION) and TIGHTENS THE CHEST. She feels that her RESPIRATORY PASSAGE IS BEING OBSTRUCTED, there is PALPITATION and the patient LOOKS PALE. She is also SWEATING and has SHORTNESS OF BREATH. She may FAINT and fall but there is neither loss of consciousness nor convulsions. There is MARKED DIMINISHED MUSCULAR TONE with COLD CLAMMY EXTREMITIES. The frequency of the attack varies. It may occur daily or even once a week. Most do not give a precipitating or aggravating cause. The attack may appear during light work or even at rest. The duration of the attack also varies. It may disappear after a short rest, or last up to hours. (I have seen one patient being bedridden for days after an attack.) These patients also have MULTIPLE PHYSICAL COMPLAINTS, EPIGASTRIC PAIN not unlike that of peptic ulcer, HEADACHE, stimulating migraine, etc. . . . In addition, the patient would almost always complain of SLEEP DISTURBANCES. . . . (Emphasis in original.)

These wide-ranging signs and symptoms have been gathered under the label *lolo mai*. According to the report, many members of Tongan society recognize the condition, which has led to this documentation of diagnostic features. However, once acknowledged, the condition becomes established as a sickness type and may have a short or long "sickness life." This may partly depend on whether western medical practice accepts the lay diagnostic label or redefines the syndrome. Already there are moves to alter the definition and absorb it into existing western images of sickness.

> I cannot help but feel this *"lolo mai"* syndrome or neurosis (whatever one would call it) is peculiar to Tongans. As it has been seen, it was hard to put a definite diagnosis for it includes a number of neurotic entities such as depression, anxiety, hypochondriasis and not to forget of course, the malingerers. No wonder then, that his condition is (as in most neurotic disorders) very difficult to manage.

Such sick people are "managed" with exercises and drugs through the psychiatric clinic.

THERAPY

Therapy as the application of a remedy is not the beginning, the middle, or the end of the healing process. The moments of the healing act consist of identifying the problem, taking action, redefining the problem, explanation, action, further explanation, and so on, until the problem has been resolved. In this section I present only the general types of Tongan therapy and limit the discussion to contemporary remedies which I observed or were described to me.

Massage

Massage is frequently used as therapy in traditional healing schemes. Massaging the whole body, or parts of the body, is an important medium of human communication; it provides a personal, supportive mode of relating to the ailing individual. Through the act of massage, empathetic understanding is directed from the healer to the sick. Here physiotherapy and psychotherapy are intimately linked and often inseparable.

Tongans recognize the influence of massage upon the sick person who is experiencing pain. A young man with a septic ulcer of the leg commented, "Often you cannot sleep because there is so much pain. You go to the right healer and they massage and you fall asleep. When you wake the pain is gone." Massage is experienced as a positive, relaxing therapy, and the sick person, weary from pain, frequently enters a deep sleep after a massage. This revitalization diminishes the pain, a result that has been observed in both Tongan and western practice.

Massage is applied with one finger, several fingers, the finger(s) and thumb, the hand(s), or the ball of the foot, depending on the kind of complaint being treated. Use of the foot, for example, is thought to be preferable in cases where care must be taken to prevent bruising.

There are three forms of massage in Tongan healing practice: *fotofota, tolotolo,* and *amoamo.* The first type of massage, *fotofota,* is the form of massage familiar to most westerners: the whole hand is used in a squeezing action, and it thus requires the most strength. *Fotofota* is used mainly for muscular aches and strains, or for massaging the *āvanga* from a possessed person's body.

1st Woman.	*Fotofota* is used, say, for *mafili* [a *fasi* disorder involving strained neck muscles]. You may have a sore neck on one side and need to be massaged for maybe a week. But also the *faitoʻo* may grind up *ʻuhi* leaves in a coconut shell with water and may massage with this medicine and some Tongan oil.
2nd Woman.	Also for *āvanga* the *faitoʻo* will use *fotofota* and *tolotolo,* massaging from the head downward, like this, to the feet. The method depends on the *faitoʻo*.
3rd Woman.	Maybe for the backache too, the *fotofota*.

Tolotolo uses a more stroking action, applying the palm of the hand with considerable pressure. This "pushing" effect is usually conducted in a lateral direction. *Tolotolo* may be used in conjunction with *fotofota* (where appropriate, all forms of massage can be so combined), and it is also used to treat such disorders as abdominal troubles, bladder and bowel complaints, and to massage the uterus to promote fertility.

Amoamo is a more gentle technique using a stroking action with a rotating or sliding movement. It is often extremely soothing, helping the sick person fall asleep. It can be used for such disorders as headache, *mata fa* (a stye in the eye), *mavae'ua* in babies, and general eye, ear, nose, and throat complaints. One example of the latter is the treatment of *ngalo'afu*:

> The lump is in the throat. This sickness is often in families [persisting through several generations]. Or it may come from eating salty food or sweet food or fatty food, so that the person with *ngalo'afu* is not to eat the food that caused it. They are given the massage, down the side of the throat. If the *ngalo'afu* is not treated, it may obstruct the throat and the person may die.

In Tongan society, *amoamo* is reportedly the only form of massage that is accompanied by the verbal act of *laulau*. *Laulau* is a form of incantation "said" inwardly by the healer so that it is inaudible to the sick person. It is considered the secret knowledge of the healer. One healer gave this example: "Say a person is choking, the *faito'o* will say something like 'Choke, pity on the person that chokes. Whatever he chokes on, fall. Give strength to the person that chokes. Whatever he chokes on, fall.'" The actual *laulau* used is seldom revealed to others. Not all healers practice it, though Tongans believe that many do, especially in cases where objects, such as a fish bone, have become lodged in the body. Today Christian prayers are sometimes used in addition to, or instead of, *laulau*.

Massage can be applied as a therapy, or part of a therapy, for any type of Tongan sickness. In cases of *āvanga* the massage can be both vigorous and soothing, and it can be applied to the whole body or a part of the body, such as the head. For *hangatāmaki* and *mahaki* the massage is usually confined to the affected part of the body and is often limited to *amoamo*, so that the inflammation or swelling of the body tissue is not aggravated. For *fasi* conditions the type of massage chosen is also governed by the complaint. One Tongan reported several episodes of backache, which were diagnosed as a *fasi* disorder and to which all three types of massage were applied, along with herbal remedies. Individuals suffering from *fasi* disorders will often return for treatment once or twice a day, and the therapy may last for several weeks or, in an extreme case, several years.

In cases of fracture, massage, manipulation, and herbal remedies are often combined. The manipulation of a fracture is performed gently but firmly, slowly working the bones back into alignment. In deciding how long to massage or how quickly to manipulate the fracture, the healer is frequently guided by the degree of pain experienced by the injured person. Some healers will apply ice, where it is occasionally available, to numb or partially anesthetize the area prior to the manipulation.

In a case I observed involving a fractured rib, the healer applied warmed Tongan oil[9] in conjunction with *amoamo,* then *tolotolo,* then *amoamo* again. Following the massage, the healer removed the excess oil from the skin with a steam towel (a strip of toweling soaked in boiling water and wrung dry), and it was explained to me that the hot cloth encourages the blood to flow after the massage has broken down any blood clot in the area.

Medicines

The principal Tongan medicines are called *vai* and *vali.* Vai means "water," hence the *vai faitoʻo* are fluid medicines with water as the main transporting substance. *Vali* are ointments, creams, and poultices. A healer explained the composition of these medicines:

> In most of the traditional medicines there are only one or two herbs used for each. One of the herbs is the active herb—*tamotamo, uhi,* and so on. The second or perhaps third herb has no medicinal value for the cure but is called *fakafāmili.* It accompanies the active one and acts as a sweetener or flavoring, but not like sugar-sweet. It covers the nasty flavor of the active ingredient. Tongan healers know that only one is the active ingredient. They know, too, that too many herbs mixed together will neutralize each other, cancel each other out.

Traditional medicines are thus distinguished from what this healer disdainfully referred to as "the modern *vai haka,*" which are "lots of leaves, boiled up and put in bottles to sell."

The *vai* medicines are used more frequently in healing practice than the ointments, so I shall concentrate on their uses. There are three forms of *vai:* the infusion *(vai mafana),* the decoction *(vai haka),* and the macerate *(vai momoko).*

In one case I heard described a *vai mafana* (lit. "warm water") was used to cure a person possessed by a spirit.

> We collected several of the *lautolu* and *lauʻuhi* leaves and placed them in a tin with boiling water. It was used [as an inhalation] by covering the person with a blanket. But we could also have used it to smear on the walls of the house, or hung the leaves up at the window or door. Also [the leaves] could have been wrapped in a cloth and put in the corner of the room. They would have chased away the spirits too. This medicine has a strong smell. The spirit hates it too.

As this speaker indicates, the herbs can be used in a variety of ways and be effective in cases of *āvanga.* Usually, a *vai* is also required in cases of spirit possession. A *faito'o āvanga* may paint or smear the possessed person's body with the preparation, massaging it into the body. The *vai* may also be used as a *tulu'i* 'drops'.

The *vai haka* (lit. "boiled water") decoctions are prepared not by boiling leaves or bark but by immersing them in hot or boiled water and then leaving them to cool. The ingredients are squeezed out, and the juice is applied to the affected part of the sick person's body. Some Tongans said the juice could be drunk if so prescribed by the healer. Others added that *vai haka* are used in cases of *āvanga* and are applied as described above.

The *vai momoko* or macerate appears to be in common use and is made by marinating medicinal herbs in cold water. The herbs are then squeezed out, and the juice is drunk or applied to the body. The traditional method of squeezing or straining medicines uses a coconut mesh or spathe called *kaka*. While this method is still practiced, today a clean (often white) cloth is sometimes used, or unbleached *tapa* called *la'i feta'aki*.

In addition to being consumed or massaged onto the body exterior, a *vai* can be applied in other ways as well. *Po* is a technique of dabbing the *vai* (or any wet preparation) onto a wound or burn. *Puhi* is another technique of administering a *vai* to a burn; it can also be used with a baby. "The medicine is blown or squirted from the mouth and is fairly commonly used. A mother may chew medicinal leaves and blow the juice into the open mouth of her child if the child has an inflamed mouth." *Vai* are also administered in the form of drops *(tulu'i)* and applied to the mouth, nose, ears, or eyes. *Tulu'i* is frequently used in cases of *āvanga,* where the medicine is said to be effective in driving the spirit away. A form of *tulu'i* called *fakatafe* is applied to ailments like boils or infected cuts; in these cases a heated stone is wrapped with medicinal leaves and the juice which exudes is dropped directly onto the wound or boil.

Vali (lit. "to smear or paint") are ointments, poultices, or creams. They are traditionally prepared by the healer chewing the leaves; today, however, herbs and bark are often ground with a stone. Occasionally, the leaves are simply warmed or steamed over a fire and applied directly to a wound.

There are numerous other preparations and techniques for treating sickness. A list of specific cures is potentially limitless. One Tongan told me,

> I remember my father had a headache that would not go away. The healer used a short brush of coconut fiber, like what we use in making our brooms. This was used to hammer a shark's tooth to make small holes, about ten or so, in his forehead. This was to let the blood out. His headache went away after a few days.

Other treatments include gargles and mouthwashes, the burning of coconut spathes for eye ailments, and staring at sticks for certain kinds of eye complaints. Medicines can be prepared from fruits as well as from leaves and bark. A preliminary medicine *(vai 'a 'ahi)* can be given as a test to assess the sick person's condition and determine the direction of further treatment. In some cases a medicine may have to be taken by the healer as well as by the sick person.

CONCLUSION

Perhaps contrary to expectation, traditional Tongan healing practices have not decreased since the introduction of western medicine but instead have developed alongside it. This is in part because of the categorical separation of western sicknesses from Tongan ones; the dual classification system suggests that western medicine, largely confined to its own sphere, is unlikely to readily displace or absorb the traditional Tongan healing practices. The admixture of Tongan, western, and other introduced healing methods has given rise to a peculiarly Tongan adaptation, one which reveals what is currently relevant to the Tongan people.

While the total array of sickness events experienced by Tongans can be classified into certain general types, the treatment of specific cases depends on individual, and sometimes idiosyncratic, interpretations. What Tongans understand about sickness and therapy (in a word, what they consider to be meaningful) will determine their decisions and actions during any particular sickness event. Thus, treating Tongans, or any people from a nonwestern culture, is not simply a matter of providing medication or surgery, with perhaps a translation of a few sickness terms. Rather, it involves dealing with an extensive range of meanings reflecting a fundamentally different worldview. Not only are the emic categories different but there is a qualitative difference in the whole sickness experience of each cultural group. Furthermore, Kleinman's argument (1980, Epilogue) impressing the need for clinical social scientists to interpret "cross-cultural illness realities" as a contribution to the redefinition of the medical model and, more immediately, as an expansion of the clinical competence of the western health professional, is supported by the findings of this study.

NOTES

I wish to thank the Medical Research Council of New Zealand for providing funds for this research in 1979–80. My thanks also to the Tongan government for permission to conduct this research. I am also indebted to the staff at Vaiola hospital, Tupou Posesi Fanua, Atolo and Sela Tu'inukuafe, Futa Helu, Louisa

Ofamo'oni, Tavi (Preben Kauffmann), Epeli Hau'ofa, and especially Semisi and 'Ofa Koloi. I also owe gratitude to all the Tongans who participated in this study.

1. The introduction of western medical ideas has been gradual. The missionary movement was perhaps the first western influence on the healing activities of the people; the second was the inauguration of the Department of Health after the world influenza epidemic of 1918–19, which killed eighteen-hundred Tongans, that is 8 percent of the population. This was in the first year of the eighteen-year-old Queen Sālote's reign. A wireless station was established in Nuku'alofa in 1920 and in Vava'u, in the north, in 1925 and has since become a major avenue for promoting western health values. Telephones were first introduced in 1919 and initially allowed the more affluent in Nuku'alofa immediate access to western health personnel. In 1929 the Fiji School of Medicine began to train selected members of Tongan society as assistant medical practitioners. By 1979 there were twenty-eight western-trained medical officers and thirteen medical assistants active throughout the Kingdom.

In 1979 the World Health Organization financed a training program with the objective of providing western-trained health personnel for the more remote regions of Tonga. These Tongan health officers are expected to act as liaison between the people, the traditional healers *(faito'o)*, and the western medical practitioners located in the four hospitals in Vava'u (Ngu), Ha'apai (Niu'ui), Tongatapu (Vaiola), and 'Eua (Niu'eiki).

2. Dingwall 1976 cites the example of South American Indians in whom dyschronic spirochetosis gives rise to spotty skin pigmentation; those without the discoloration—that is, healthy individuals by western standards—are ineligible for marriage.

3. For a list of pregnancy *tapu*s, see Parsons 1981a.

4. This opposes Schwartz's notion of a "hierarchy of curative resort." See also Parsons 1984.

5. Martin 1827; Collocott 1923; Gifford 1929.

6. See Parsons 1984 for accounts of loneliness, isolation, and deviance in relation to spirit attack.

7. A study conducted in liaison with McGill University (report issued in 1979) showed an increase in psychiatric illness in Tonga. Recent Department of Health reports show a similar pattern of redefining "disturbed" behavior among Tongans and classifying them as "psychiatric."

8. Exhumation is possible in Tonga, and it is performed without due ceremony. The Department of Health requires that permission be obtained "in case the deceased died of an infectious disease [and] ask that only one person, usually the affected person, open the grave." In practice, however, the Tongans I spoke with did not seem to be concerned with following such a procedure, and indeed most did not know of the Department's request.

9. According to Weiner 1971, the Tongan oil used in massage is prepared by pounding the endocarp of the nuts of *Aleurites moluccana* with the leaves or flowers of *Melastoma denticulatum, Decaspermum fruticosum, Cinnamonum* Spp., and *Coleus amboinicus,* to which is added the oil of grated coconut. The

Tongan oil is compressed and strained from this mixture on the following day. When I spoke to the person in the king's household who prepares Tongan oil for the royal family, however, she indicated that she uses many ingredients and makes many types of Tongan oil, both for massage and for body decoration and perfumery. Her recipes are part of her own esoteric knowledge.

6

Contemporary Healing Practices in East Futuna

Bruce Biggs

For some time, as part of wider ethnolinguistic research, I have been inquiring into the nature of local healing practices on the island of Futuna in the Horne Islands, which should not be confused with the Futuna in the New Hebrides (now Vanuatu). Linguists distinguish the Polynesian languages spoken on the two islands as East Futunan and West Futunan. The Horne Islands, Futuna and 'Alofi, are two small but high islands separated by a deep channel about half a mile wide. Futuna has an area of 25 square miles and a highest point of 2500 feet above sea level. Its neighbor, 'Alofi, is 11 square miles in area and 1200 feet high. Together with Wallis Island ('Uvea), about 120 miles to the northeast, the Horne Islands comprise a self-governing overseas territory of France, Les Iles des Wallis et Futuna, situated between Fiji and Samoa.

I first saw the Horne Islands from the deck of a liner traveling south from San Francisco to Auckland. The weather was bad and from design or accident the eastern side of 'Alofi loomed out of the overcast close enough for us to see people walking on the beautiful and usually deserted beach of that island, which has no permanent residents. My imagination was caught by the sight and I vowed that I would go there some day. I redeemed my vow more than a decade later when, in the company of Douglas Yen, ethnobotanist at the Bernice P. Bishop Museum, Honolulu, I spent thirty days on Futuna.

LINGUISTIC, CULTURAL, AND BOTANICAL AFFINITIES OF EAST FUTUNA

The population of Futuna is Polynesian, speaking East Futunan, a language of the subgroup called Samoic-Outlier. Almost all of the three thousand or so people living on the island are familiar with the closely

Contemporary Healing Practices in East Futuna

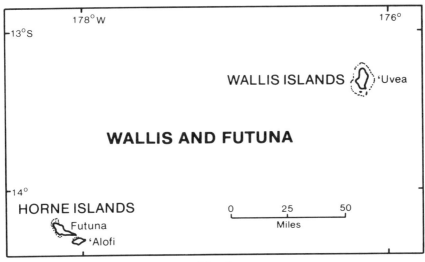

Map 5

related, but not quite mutually intelligible, East 'Uvean language spoken on Wallis Island. Like other Polynesian languages, East Futunan is phonologically simple. An alphabet of just sixteen symbols is sufficient to notate all phonemic contrasts. All Futunans are literate in the vernacular language, and I use their orthography except that I mark glottal stops and long vowels whereas they normally leave these phonemic distinctions unmarked.

It has recently been established that Futuna has been settled for more than two thousand years (Kirch 1976). There is some evidence that, up until first European contact, Futuna was in at least sporadic contact with Cikobia and Naqelelevu, the easternmost islands of the Fijian Group (Biggs and Biggs 1975, 11–14). Linguistic evidence suggests fairly recent influence from Samoa, and there has been much influence on the language, especially in historic times, from Wallis Island, which was itself extensively influenced by Tongan colonization, probably in the sixteenth century. Direct contacts with Tonga are also attested by tradition and historical evidence from the eighteenth century on. Since the mid-nineteenth century contact between Wallis Island and Futuna has been frequent. During the past fifty years there has been much contact with New Caledonia and Vanuatu. Most of the adult Futunan population has visited New Caledonia, at least.

Botanically speaking, Futuna is part of a Fijian region comprising the archipelagoes between the New Hebrides and Samoa, and including Rotuma and Wallis Island:

Of the presently known 248 species of vascular plants in the Horne and Wallis Islands, 170 appear to be indigenous. Of these 125 are wide-spread, at least in the Pacific, but a considerable number of these (19) do not extend east of the Fijian region. . . . 45 species indigenous to the Horne and Wallis Islands are limited to the Fijian region. Although many of these occur in both Fiji and Samoa, relationships with the latter archipelago appear stronger than with the former. (St. John and Smith 1971, 315)

RESEARCH METHODS

"It is a matter of common agreement among modern anthropological field-workers that an account of the institutions of a native people should contain some description of the methods by which the information was obtained" (Firth 1936, 3). Firth goes on to list the points that should be made clear, which include the nature and duration of the contact, the language used to gather the information and whether it was paid for; whether it describes current or obsolete practice, and whether it represents direct observation or hearsay. The range of observations upon which generalizations are made should also be indicated.

It would also be generally agreed by anthropologists that the contact between the investigator and informants should be of reasonable duration and intimacy, the contact language should be that carrying the cultural institutions being investigated, and a reasonable amount of direct observation should be involved. This has not always been the case, of course. My teacher, Ralph Piddington, used to paint a humorous picture of the nineteenth-century anthropologist on a brief trip to the field, lining up the local population and questioning them through an interpreter after having failed to gain from the colonial administrator any more information on local manners and customs than that the former were nonexistent and the latter beastly.

Nonanthropologists, and perhaps even some anthropologists, do not always comply with Firth's requirements when doing research in Polynesia, and for certain purposes that may not matter too much. If you are a pharmaceutical chemist interested only in what plants are used for whatever maladies, you can probably get useful information from someone who knows *your* language, or even through an interpreter, and in fairly quick time.

If, however, you want to know what people *do* in healing practice, rather than what they say they do, you will have to be what the anthropologists call a participant observer, and this usually requires a substantial period of living among your subjects. If you want to understand fully the ideas of sickness and health that underlie your healer's practices, his categories of disease, and the specialized vocabulary of his profession, you must work in *his* language, not yours, because while you may, eventually, get to understand what he tells you in his language, and translate it into something that can be compared with western ideas on the same topic, there is no way that your informant, perfect though his English may be, can do that for you. His very use of English will mask and obscure your topic of investigation. At least that is how it seems to me.

Anthropologists have, I feel, tended to say too little about communication problems in their work. Those who have not worked in the vernacular language of their people tend to gloss over the fact that they have not met one of the ideal requirements of their discipline. There has been the occasional apologia asserting that only a superficial knowledge of the local tongue is really required, and that it may be acquired easily (Mead 1939). But this assertion would not meet with general agreement. Those who claim to use the vernacular language mainly, or exclusively, vary widely in their statements as to how long it took to attain the necessary competence. Firth "abandoned entirely" the use of a *lingua franca* after only three weeks in the field, but such a case is exceptional, and he had prior knowledge of a related Polynesian language.

Although we all learn one language perfectly, we vary enormously in our ability to acquire another. It is clear that some languages are harder to learn than others. Few of the many anthropologists who have worked in the New Guinea Highlands seem to have worked exclusively in local languages; on the other hand, fieldworkers in Polynesia usually become speakers of the vernacular concerned.

My own experience differed from most. I did not use English at all on my first trip to Futuna because on that French island I met no English speakers among the Futunans. Not speaking French, I was forced to use Polynesian from the beginning. Helped by my knowledge of Maori and other Polynesian languages, and armed with Grezel's *Dictionnaire Futunien-Français,* I was able to converse haltingly in Futunan by the end of a month, by which I mean I was able to ask my carefully worked out questions and, if lucky, understand the answers. (I have never found that I understand a language better than I can speak it, as people often claim to do.)

Fieldworkers today have, in the tape recorder, an inestimable advantage over earlier generations of fieldworkers. My Sony TC800, a model that has never been surpassed for the working anthropologist, was kept switched on throughout informant sessions. Between sessions I worked over what informants really had said, and framed new questions for next time. The early tapes, on which informants and investigator both reveal the excitement of initial contact with an unfamiliar culture, can still be studied and, extraordinarily, each new audition seems to reveal some nuance in the informant's answer, or some hitherto unnoticed comment by a voice in the background. I feel sorry for the fieldworker of earlier days whose only evidence for any incident are his notebooks, frozen references to first impressions.

When writing up the results of his research, the fieldworker in an exotic culture faces a special problem in convincing others that things are really as he says. He cannot send his critics to their laboratories to repeat experiments for themselves. His reports must carry their own conviction. Traditionally this has been attained by two techniques characteristic of, but not confined to, anthropological monographs. In the "case study" approach a detailed account of actual happenings substitutes for descriptions of experiments, and "direct quotation" of informants' responses aids the conviction that conclusions are based on observed data. I will use both techniques in what follows, sparingly for reasons of space, but sufficiently, I hope, to convince readers that any conclusions drawn are at least plausible ones.

PAST AND PRESENT RESEARCH ON PLANT MEDICINE IN FUTUNA

There has been little, if any, previous study of indigenous medical practices on Futuna. Edwin G. Burrows, who spent four months on the island in 1932, has this to say:

> The old Futunan practices of healing are still in general use. Even some of the supernatural beliefs about disease and remedy have survived, though weakened now, and usually dissociated from the names of pagan gods. (Burrows 1936, 113)

Burrows mentions the use of massage in healing, and the scoring of flesh to treat filarial swelling, but says that plant medicines are the most frequently used of all Futunan remedies. One man told him that all the leaves of Futuna were used as remedies. Burrow's comments remain true, though he gives little or no detail of the extensive use of plant medicine that must have been flourishing in Futuna in his time. Pagan gods are now disavowed, and all medicine is practiced in the name of Christianity, though not, as far as I am aware, with the approval of the church. In some cases illness itself is associated with Satana, the devil, or more generally with supernatural beings called *temonio,* who may be thought of as the spirits of the dead.

Again Burrows gives little specific information about concepts of health and sickness, though he mentions the belief, also found in Fiji, that a child should have yaws if it is to thrive (Burrows 1936, 114). He also recounts an incident where efforts were made to catch a malevolent spirit that was believed to have been the cause of a man suffering a fall from a tree. He mentions that Futunans appeared to expect instant results from medicine, and if such were not forthcoming, another remedy would be tried. This has implications for a theory which tries to capture the Futunan view of sickness, as we shall see.

In 1969 Douglas Yen, ethnobotanist at the Bishop Museum, and I spent a month on Futuna. Yen collected specimens of fifty-seven plants used medicinally, as well as seventy-six not so used. All of the plants were identified by Harold St. John of the Bishop Museum and Albert C. Smith of the University of Massachusetts (St. John and Smith 1971). Since 1969 I have made several further trips to Futuna and spent a total of about seven months on the island; in addition I have had two months in Noumea continuing my inquiries with Futunans resident there, and Futunan friends have stayed for several months with my wife and me at our home in Auckland.

Any adult Futunan may practice *faito'o* 'healing'. Burrows reported that nearly every man was the proprietor of at least one remedy and some had as many as thirty. But all practitioners I have met, other than specialists in massage, were women. It is commonly said that men, too, are healers, and many, perhaps all, men practice massage, which is likely to be used in addition to medicine in many treatments. Knowledge of the medicinal uses of at least some plants is common to all women, but those who are considered to be skilled healers are generally those who are old enough, middle-aged or better, to be called *finematu'a*. Practitioners generally claim to specialize in the use of one or a few medicines, and are called on when it is thought that their particular expertise is appropriate. For example, I have seen two cases of treatment for ghost sickness (*'āvaga*) in the same village, one in 1971 and the other in 1980. In both cases the same *finematu'a* was called on.

THE NATURE OF TRADITIONAL MEDICAL TREATMENT

Infusions of plant material, massage, and prayer are the main ingredients of traditional healing in Futuna. As illness is caused either naturally or by malignant spirits, and not by previous sinful or unsocial behavior of the patient, no prolonged psychoanalytic type of inquiry is held, nor is there found in Futuna any supportive type of counseling such as occurs in current Maori healing practice, for example.

Burrows mentions that massage is used for many ailments. *Fakasolosolo* is the general word for massage. *Milimili* is a gentle stroking or anointing with oil or other unguent, and *amoamo* is a gentle fondling or touching. *Lusilusi* involves firm kneading of the muscles, and *lomilomi*, pressing down with the full weight of the masseur's body. Some forms of massage can be very painful, especially if performed by a strong man. Different practitioners favor different massage styles, one using the heels of the hands, another using thumbs and fingertips to probe the muscles where they pass over bones. This latter, called *kinikini* or *faiʻua,* is a particularly painful style. For backache the patient, lying prone, may be walked on by the masseur. I was told that it was appropriate for the masseur to be of the same sex as the patient but observed instances where this was not the case.

As Douglas Yen was collecting specimens of plants Futunans said they used in healing, it was natural for me to begin my own investigations by asking, independently, the uses *(ʻaoga)* of various plants, rather than starting, for example, with an inquiry into kinds of illnesses. The flora of Futuna is rich and all Futunans, including children, are very knowledgeable about it. Moreover, at least as far as women are concerned, the medicinal uses of plants are of prime interest. A plant that has no medicinal use may be dismissed with the scornful comment "it has no use" *(leʻai sona ʻaoga).* It is tempting to say that the plant, as medicine, rather than the ailment as disease category, is of prime importance in Futunan thought on these matters.

An initial inquiry as to the medicinal use of a plant generally receives a formula-like reply that begins with the name of the plant and a brief and essentially technical statement of its use. Such replies tend to be recited as if they have been learned by heart, almost chanted, though it is not implied that each informant will give exactly the same formula:

Q. What is the use of *Canavalia maritima?*
A. The *Canavalia maritima:* it makes a potion for a woman in labor.

These formulae leave out a great deal of information that we would expect to find in, say, a cooking recipe, or a prescription for some home remedy. It is unusual for any dose to be mentioned, or for the method of making the medicine from the plant to be described. At first sight such omissions seem to make these prescriptions, if we may call them such, of little value as a guide to how Futunans actually use these plants medicinally. But they are not quite as inexplicit as they appear to be. Medicine is made in a limited number of ways, and often simply naming the type of medicine—for example, *vai* 'infusion of plant material in water', *mili* 'liniment', *tuluʻi* 'drops'—will indicate to the initiate how it is to be prepared and used. Also such words from the general vocabulary as *valu* 'scrape, scrapings', *mama* 'chew', *kisu* 'spit out', *kofu* 'wrap up', *soa* 'friend' have more specialized technical meanings in a medical context and when so used denote a specific procedure.

At some later date, after I had worked over the tapes and made sure that I understood the answers received so far, I would take up the topic again, eliciting more detailed information.

Q. The *Canavalia maritima:* when a woman is ill, prepare the leaves and drink. Is that right?
A. Yes.
Q. What kind of illness?
A. Stomach pain.
Q. Woman or girl?
A. Both women and girls the same.
Q. And men?
A. No. This potion is for women who dwell and their stomach pains. The root of the pain is that it comes together with her period; that is why men do not use that medicine. The name of the illness is *mataki loto*. It is illness in the stomach; and that illness can stem from a woman having given birth. When her labor is over her stomach may pain. Then mix the medicine.

Dosage is not critical in the case of liniments and drops. With potions I believe it is usual to drink all that is prepared at one time (about half a cup in the cases I have seen) as a single dose, except for a small amount retained to be used as a liniment in the case of some medicines. This residue is called *suʻa*. The strength of the "infusion" of course still remains unspecified, but this may be deliberate. While most Futunan women can recite the uses of many medicinal plants, few of them practice medicine in anything but a perfunctory way, and of these few each has her own specialty or specialties. The specialized knowledge includes information as to the exact number of leaves to be used in an infusion, for example. The best number varies from specialist to specialist, though it seems general that leaves from the plant are counted in pairs *(soa)* and not taken singly. This kind of information is, in a sense, esoteric, and as such is not included in the casual recitation of prescriptions.

The reader of descriptions of medicinal practices among folk societies may well be tempted to ask how general the practices described are within the society, and whether recipes persist or are continually being changed. Perhaps medical practices are quite idiosyncratic to each practitioner? It is not that a remedy used by a single healer is any less legitimate than one practiced by all; nor is a newly devised prescription less valid than one that has been used for generations. But such information is relevant, and is all too often missing from reports on folk healing. It is surely worth knowing whether a putative remedy is widely regarded as being effective or not, whether perhaps the informant, sincerely or otherwise, is actually putting you wrong. There are fairly obvious ways of avoiding some of the traps. Information given in public is subject to correction by those listening; if given in private it can be rechecked at a later date with the same informant or another.

In the absence of earlier information it is impossible to know whether or not given recipes are traditional. For Futuna, Burrows, the only previous investigator, mentions just three specific plant remedies: *milo* bark for filarial enlargement of the scrotum; *valovalo* leaves to make a potion for sore throat; and the same used as an unguent for *mili avaga* (sic). Burrows, who knew that *'āvaga* means marriage but not that it also means "ghost sickness," thought that *mili avaga* might be a disease having something to do with the sexual organs or functions.

Forty years after Burrows I observed for myself *valovalo (Premna taitensis)* leaves being chewed up and used in the treatment of ghost sickness, but I did not hear that they were used as a potion for sore throat. I was told that *milo* bark was the part of the tree that is used medicinally, but not for the purpose mentioned by Burrows.

The appendix to this paper sets out most of the information I have gathered about the plants used medicinally on Futuna. Most of this is set down as an English translation of the words of the informants, but in some cases it is supported with vernacular text which will be intelligible (or nearly so) to speakers of other Polynesian languages. In most cases it will be observed that there is a high degree of agreement among informants as to the uses of each plant. In cases where there is disagreement there may have been misunderstanding on my part. Better eliciting might have made it clear that different parts of the plant were being referred to by different persons, or that several conditions were in fact treated by the same medicine because they are considered to be part of the same illness. For example "relapse medicine" *(vai kita)* may be used as a potion, a liniment, and as eardrops to treat fever, body pain, and headache, all of which are regarded as symptoms of different named manifestations of the sickness. In some cases there may have been reluctance on the part of an informant to admit to certain kinds of medical practice, such as the cure of spirit sickness, reference to which is disapproved by the church, or the use of abortifacients, which is believed to be illegal.

SOME FUTUNAN SICKNESS CATEGORIES

To be well or healthy is *mālōlō*. To be ill is *masaki*. *Masaki* may be part of the normal order of things, or it may be caused by supernatural influences, in which case it is called *'āvaga* and has its own treatment. The following, from an interview conducted in English in Noumea, illustrates that ghost sickness is put into a quite different category from other maladies:

Q. What about *'āvaga?*
A. *'Āvaga* is *temonio* [ghosts].
Q. If you get *manava* [stomach pain], that's not *'āvaga?*
A. No. That's just *masaki.*
Q. If you had *'āvaga* would you go to the French doctor?
A. No, because he don't *know!* Every time, if somebody's like that, when he go to see the doctor he give some medicine. Doesn't *do* nothing. So we go to see someone who knows, who do the *'āvaga.*

There is a fairly clear distinction between sickness *(masaki)* and injury *(lavea).* Among natural illnesses, one that assumes disproportionate status is called *kita. Kita* takes various forms and has several subvarieties; its one invariable feature is that it succeeds apparent recovery from an earlier illness. We may translate *kita* as "relapse" and its medicine *vai kita* as "relapse medicine," while remembering that to Futunans it is a definite category of disease, caused in their view by premature return to hard manual work after being ill.

Symptoms of particular diseases are not much studied by Futunans. Certain symptoms are, it is true, recognized because they are obvious. Pain in various body parts, fever, chill, suppuration, swelling, headache, diarrhoea, and delirium are all recognized but may occur in more than one kind of *masaki,* which is to say they may receive more than one kind of treatment, though the last-named would be prima facie evidence of *'āvaga* or spirit sickness.

In general the diagnosis of non-obvious disease appears to be decided by the medicine which cures it. This explains a tendency reported by Burrows—to want to try a new medicine when the first one has no immediate beneficial effect. It is not until the medicine has worked that diagnosis is confirmed. In line with this thinking, a disease and its treatment often have the same name—for example, *'āvaga* refers to spirit sickness and its treatment, and *kita* is often used to refer to the medicine as well as the sickness itself. There is general difficulty in getting detailed descriptions of symptoms which might determine the nature of a sickness, but there is great willingness on the part of Futunans to talk about the medicines themselves.

Nevertheless, it is possible for certain named disease categories to put together a description of symptoms that would influence the diagnosis. I discuss three of these briefly; all of them seem to me not to translate into western disease entities. The combinations of physical symptoms and external circumstances used by Futunans would often not be considered relevant by us. For example, it is clear that the *finematu'a* who chided her patient for leaving his window open at night, thus encouraging entry by spirits of the dead, had taken account of this open window in her diagnosis of "ghost sickness." The open window would probably not be considered relevant by a modern physician, though it might have been considered by his forebears who took night-air miasmas into account.

Similarly, the factor of relapse is not taken to be a defining criterion for a disease category in western medicine as it is, apparently, for the Futunan category called *kita*. Finally, as far as I have been able to ascertain, the sickness called *toka'ala* has, as its defining symptom, belly pain or other untoward complications following childbirth, which would not define a single ailment in western medicine.

'ĀVAGA, THE SICKNESS CAUSED BY GHOSTS

In its classic form *'āvaga* is characterized by abnormal behavior, as in delirium, or certain phychoses. It is said that a person who is *'āvea*, which is to say afflicted by *'āvaga*, behaves "as if his body were very strong but he had lost his senses." It is clear, from a number of cases described to me, that *'āvaga* often follows some personal crisis, such as the loss of a close relative. It is not always associated with irrational behavior, as we shall see. It seems likely that any illness with no obvious cause may, in certain circumstances, be treated as a case of *'āvaga*.

In Futunan thought *'āvaga* is due to the ill will of the spirits *(temonio)* who are variously thought of as the spirits of the forest, or of the recent dead, or as the devil *(Satana)*. It is considered dangerous to go to places where *temonio* are, and especially dangerous to behave disrespectfully there. You may actually be attacked physically by a *temonio*, though more subtle forms of affliction are more usual. One informant had this to say of *'āvaga*:

> It is called *'āvea* [carried off] here in Futuna. Characteristically a man is struck by a ghost in the forest. There are many ghosts in Futuna. . . . They say that though Christianity may grow stronger those things do not disappear. . . . But I do not believe that one is struck. It is the blood. Just the blood descending from the head. I think this because during my life no ghost has yet appeared in the world, walking on the road, striking men. It is [because of] Christianity. It is just the blood from the head, and then the speech goes awry. The one afflicted has a bad headache, and speaks stupidly, because of the sickness in his head.

A man may be approached in a dream by a spirit which has taken the appearance of a close friend or associate. If the dreamer should accept food proffered by the spirit, then he will certainly sicken when he awakes. If the disguised spirit should touch any part of the dreamer's body, he will be afflicted in that part. Following is an account of a case of *'āvaga* and the treatment used.

A man dreamed that his wife, from whom he was separated at the time, had visited him. He mentioned the dream to a woman acquaintance who said, "That was not your wife but a spirit. Moreover, you should expect such visitations if you insist on sleeping with the windows and doors open, allowing access to any spirit from the bush." Two days later, as was feared by the woman, the man became ill, vomiting and sweating, and suffering from general malaise. He took to his bed, and the woman acquaintance said, "I had better go and get an old woman [i.e. someone skilled in *faito'o*]."

The old woman, a recognized expert in the treatment of *'āvaga*, arrived and talked to the patient, warning him that if she was to treat him he must promise not to go out in the sun until he was well. If he did she would become ill herself. She also chided him, saying, "I hear that you sleep with windows open. Don't you realize that when people die their bodies are carried along the road past your house on their way to the cemetery. If you must have windows open let them be those facing the sea. Keep the ones facing the road closed."

The first part of the treatment was a prolonged and painful massage from head to toe, with thumbs and fingertips probing each muscle, especially over bones, where strong pressure could be exerted. Plain water was used instead of oil as a liniment *(mili)*. The practitioner then went away and returned later with young leaves of *valovalo (Premna taitensis)* which she took, in pairs, and made into a wad the size of a walnut. Crossing herself, she popped them into her mouth with an expression of distaste. (All *'āvaga* medicine is said to smell bad. Spirits are driven away by the unpleasant smell.) The chewed leaves were put into a cup of water. Then the massage was repeated using the medicine as *mili*, thus coating the patient with a spattering of chewed fragments of the *valovalo* leaves. The patient was warned not to wash them off until recovery was complete, which turned out to be two days later.

In a second case I observed, a young Futunan woman who had lived in Fiji for many years returned to Futuna and was working in one of the shops there. It was said that she was anxious to go back to Fiji but was unable to do so. On one occasion when the owner of the shop was giving a dinner party in the compound of the shop and the young woman was serving drinks, it was noticed that she was partaking as well as dispensing. Her behavior became erratic, apparently, and my first indication of trouble was seeing a group pursue her and proceed toward a large trough in which they proposed to duck her. I interfered and she was taken, instead, to a house and laid on a bed and restrained physically. She was talking wildly, mainly in English, and frequently repeating, "Let me go! Let me go!" referring, it seemed, to her wish to return to Fiji.

The same healer was fetched and an abbreviated version of the procedure described above was followed. At one point I was asked to leave the room as her *koga* 'parts' were about to be treated. On the following day she was back at her job in the shop, friendly and rational. The incident seemed to have attracted only mild interest.

THE LANGUAGE OF HEALING

English characteristically borrows technical vocabulary from the classical languages, except for traditional crafts, which often have native technical vocabulary. The Polynesians, however, had had little or no contact with alien languages for a couple of thousand years. Their technical language was, perforce, derived from ordinary, nonspecialized vocabulary. In ordinary speech *vai, mili, tuluʻi, kisu* mean "water," "rub," "drip," "spit out," respectively. In the context of healing they take on the technical meanings of "medicine to be drunk (potion)," "embrocation," "medicinal drops," and "spraying chewed-up medicinal leaves from the mouth," respectively. All Futunans know both the ordinary and technical meanings of such words. There is no esoteric vocabulary such as was found among the New Zealand Maori, for example. Technical metaphors are found, too, but again they are known to everyone. *Inu vai* means "drink water" but in the appropriate context it means "undergo superincision." Such metaphors are not predictable, of course, but many of them are obvious enough when known—the use of the word *fonu* 'turtle' to refer to the condition of hunchback, for example. Some are designedly cryptic, as when one says *e uʻa le tai* 'the tide is in', meaning that a hunchback is present.

Some technical words have no ordinary, nontechnical meaning. *Faitoʻo,* the word for traditional medical treatment, is one such, and the word *kita,* applied to a conceptually important kind of illness, is another. When technical words do have ordinary everyday meanings, however, the question whether the two meanings for the same form should be regarded as extensions of the same basic meaning, or whether two homonyms are involved, can be puzzling. Fairly clearly, *vai* 'water' and *vai* 'liquid' (e.g. amniotic fluid) and *vai* 'medicine' are extensions of the same meaning. But what about *ʻāvaga* 'spouse' and *ʻāvaga* 'psychosis'? Characteristically, an *ʻāvaga* attack is initiated by a spirit *(temonio)* taking the form of a person known to you, often your spouse, and appearing in a dream and trying to persuade you to accept food or other favors. My informants denied any connection between the two words.

While *ʻāvaga* meaning "spouse, to marry" is widespread in the western

Polynesian area, the meaning "ghost-sickness" is restricted to Futuna, Tonga, and 'Uvea. This is also true of *kita* 'relapse' and *faito'o* 'healing practices', which suggests that in Futuna these medical meanings are borrowings rather than natural extensions of the ordinary meanings. This in turn raises the question whether some or all of contemporary healing practices in Futuna are intrusive. Unfortunately, I did not discuss this possibility with my informants, but it may be significant that, as far as I know, early missionary accounts make little mention of the use of plant medicines in Futuna (see Burrows 1936, 115).

The converse of the homonym problem is the problem of synonyms, but it is inherently easier to solve. *Any* difference of meaning between two forms disqualifies them as synonyms, but it is the *degree* of similarity in meaning, as determined by the native speaker's intuition, that decides whether the same form should be considered as two homonyms or not. Unfortunately, one may be left unaware of problems of synonymy until one has left the field, and poring over field tapes may not solve the problems later. I have, for example, noted several terms for a condition described as "enlarged scrotum," but I neglected to enquire whether the terminological distinctions are meant to indicate different diseases, or even whether they distinguish polite versus vulgar references to the same condition.

Infusions of plant material are distinguished as potions *(vai)*, drops to be dripped into body apertures *(tulu'i)*, or liniments to be rubbed on the skin *(mili)*. The parts of plants that are used and distinguished terminologically are leaves *(lau)*, bark *(kili)*, lower trunk *(tafito)*, fruit *(fua)*, unopened buds or shoots *(muko)*, and stems or trunks *(kuaga)*.

When medicine is administered a prayer *(kole)* is said, either aloud or sotto voce, accompanied by a sign of the cross. My information is that all prayers are Christian prayers and there are no remnants of the old pagan religion practiced at present. After resisting conversion in the early 1840s, Futunans converted en masse to Christianity after the massacre of Pierre Chanel in 1841. All Futunans today are practicing Catholics.

ATTITUDES TO WESTERN MEDICINE

Futunans are practical people. For them healing is as healing does. The continuation of traditional healing practices is not accompanied by any rejection of the services offered by the French doctor and his staff at the two little hospitals maintained on the island, one in Sigave district and the other in 'Alo. Futunans can observe for themselves the often dramatically beneficial effects of antibiotics, for example, and *suki* (injection) is recognized by everyone as a legitimate and effective healing technique, one practiced by the *toketā* but not by the *faito'o*.

Those suffering serious lesions and fractures are taken to the *opitale* for treatment, and the occasional need for internal surgery is accepted, though not necessarily understood. Nevertheless, before entering hospital a patient may very well have been treated by *faito'o* previously, either in an attempt to effect a cure or simply as an appropriate preparation for entry to hospital. For example, while all births are said to take place at hospital nowadays preparatory Futunan medicines are said to be taken beforehand, and, in certain cases, after return from hospital:

> When a woman feels her pains and is going to hospital, go and fetch *Canavalia maritima*, and pound it and shred its leaves—the *Canavalia* and the *Hibiscus rosa sinensis* are the same. Bring the leaves, wrap them in a piece of cloth, pound them and mix with water and give to the woman to drink who is going to the hospital. Make it and drink it, then go to hospital. It is done to hasten the coming down of the child. After the birth obey the hospital. On returning home, if her belly pains and the blood comes badly, go and fetch Futunan medicine and drink it and the blood will come freely and the woman's belly will be alright.

Perhaps the only minor surgery that is still, occasionally, practiced at home is superincision of the penis, which all boys undergo at early adolescence. I was told that all boys from Sigave district are now superincised at the hospital, as required by the doctor, while many superincisions are still done at home in 'Alo. However, I witnessed one superincision ceremony in Sigave some years ago. The procedure did not differ significantly from that described in Burrows (1936, 61) and Gaillot (1962, 207), so I will not describe it further here.

NOTE

My friend and colleague Doug Yen made possible my first trip to Futuna, aroused my interest in Futunan plant medicine, and made the plant collection which underpins this paper and without which it could not have been written. The French people resident on Futuna on my various visits have extended the kindest hospitality to me at all times. I mention especially Mr. Garcia and his wife, who made Yen and myself welcome on our first trip, and my friend Michel Gaveau and his wife, Maliana, at whose lovely home in Somalama I stayed in January 1981. Gideon Jessop's kindness to me has always been unstinted and it was a privilege to repay his hospitality in a small way, when he and members of his family visited us in Auckland some years ago. Gideon's father, Petelo Vaka Jessop, and his mother's brother, Lavelua Keleta'ona, were both very good friends to me and I pay my respects to their memory. Finally I want to thank all the Futunans, and there are many of them, who have contributed to what little I have learned of the matter in hand, giving as freely of their knowledge as my understanding of their language would allow. *Mālō le 'alofa*. Though I was never urged to keep secret what was told to me, it is not without some misgivings that I set it down here.

APPENDIX: PHARMACOPOEIA FUTUNENSIS

Specimens of almost all of the following plants were collected by Douglas Yen on Futuna and 'Alofi in 1969 and identifications made by Harold St. John and Albert C. Smith (St. John and Smith 1971). Some preliminary information regarding the medicinal uses of each plant was obtained by Yen. The list of plants used medicinally is tentative and expected to be incomplete. Two-letter codes for informants are parenthesized.

1. *Magele (Trema orientalis)*
There is considerable inconsistency among my informants as to the medicinal uses of this plant. (IP) says that an infusion of the bark is used as a liniment and potion for backache, while a potion of unspecified use is made from the leaves. (AP) says it is used for eardrops to cure earache. (TL) says that the bark makes a potion used for mouth and throat infections *(vai pala)*.

2. *Fue (Canavalia maritima)*
(AP) (ST) (MS) (VS) (IP) say that the leaves of this creeping plant, which covers much of the foreshore of Futuna, are used to make an infusion used both as potion and liniment, for women patients only, and in the following circumstances: (a) When a woman or girl has a stomachache which "descends to her" *(ifo kiate ia)*. This latter idiom refers to sickness associated with the reproductive system. This particular condition is called *mataki loto* which might be translated as "stretched within." It is normally, but not exclusively, associated with pregnancy. (b) At the onset of labor, before the woman is taken to hospital. (c) After childbirth, if it is considered that there has not been sufficient bleeding. The infusion was referred to by all informants as a *vai fānau* 'birth potion'.

3. *'Ū (An unidentified large reedlike grass)*
According to (AP) juice is expressed from the young unexpanded leaf shoots into an injured eye. But (IP) says that the shoot, which, though soft, has a sharp point and a finely serrated edge, is used to gently scrape and probe an eye which is blind so that blood appears *(e mafiti mai le toto)* and runs away *(e 'au le toto ki tafa)*. "Then," she says, "you will see clearly" *(e kē tio mālama)*.

4. *Kala'apusi (Acalypha grandis)*
(IP): An infusion of the bark is taken for lassitude and general weakness *(gaegae)* to restore energy and strength *(makeke)*. On another occasion she said it was applied for body pains, and on yet another occasion that it was used as drops *(tulu'i)* for headache. It is not unlikely that all three statements are correct.

5. *Nonu (Morinda citrifolia)*
(AP) (ST) (IP): The fruit is chewed and the juice dripped onto the lips of children with ulcerated mouths *(gutu papala)*. (ST): a potion is made from the bark and

taken by women with stomach pains. Like *'afa, tiale,* and *pua* (q.v.) it is taken by pregnant women who do not want a child *(sē fia fai tamaliki).*

6. *Milo (Thespesia populnea)*
(AP) (MS): Crushed bark scrapings from mature trees are steeped to make a potion used for stomach pains. Others said the potion so made was for a cough (IP), "relapse medicine" *(vai kita)* (VS), or rheumatic pains (Yen).

7. *Pilo (Geniostoma samoense)*
(IP): A woman about to give birth goes and scrapes the trunk and mixes the potion and drinks, then goes and gives birth . . . mix *ifi* and *pilo* together. In your eighth month go to the woman who practices medicine; [ask her] to bring *pilo* and *ifi* for you to drink. After that go and give birth and there will be no bad aftereffects. *(Ko le fafine e teuteu fānau ti ano o valu lona kuaga, o palu, o inu, ti fano o fānau . . . e fakatasi le ifi mo le pilo o inu e koe. Ti 'oki, ti kē ano o fānau, e lē'ai se kē masaki.)*

(ST): When a woman feels her pains, then [she should] drink [a potion of] its scrapings and go to the hospital. *(E mamae le gā-ne'a o le fafine, ti inu ki lona kuaga, ti fano ki Pule'aga.)* The leaves are used for drops *(tulu'i)* for sick children.

(IP): The leaves, together with [*ma'ota*] leaves, are used to make drops *(tulu'i)* and a liniment *(mili)* for headache and feverishness, respectively. These are all used in connection with ghost sickness *('āvaga).*

8. *Ma'ota (Dysoxylum samoense)*
(IP): The leaves are used to make a liniment for inflammation and feverishness.

9. *Vī-so'a (Colubrina asiatica)*
(AP) (IP) (ST): The leaves make a potion for diarrhoea *(vai liligi).*

10. *Ola (Randia cochinchensis)*
(IP) (ST): The leaves are used to make a liniment *(mili)* for babies who are feverish and in pain.

(ST): In some cases the illness is regarded as ghost sickness *('āvaga)* and the medicine is then called *mili 'āvaga.*

11. *Tiale (Gardenia taitensis;* Tahitian gardenia)
(AP) (IP) (ST): The bark from this shrub is said to be an abortifacient.

(ST): The *tiale,* its trunk is scraped and this is the medicine that causes children to abort. The *tiale* and *nonu* are alike, and the *pua* and the *'afa.* If the pregnant woman drinks then the child will fall and die. The woman who does not want children. *(Ko le tiale, ko lona kuaga, e valu, ko le vai fakatō tamaliki. Tatau le tiale mo le nonu. Mo le pua mo le 'afa. E inu le fafine e faitama, ti vilo lana tama, o mate. Ko le fafine sē fia fai tamaliki.)*

(IP): The woman who is pregnant, and resents her pregnancy, then fetches the *tiale* and scrapes it, and mixes it with *nonu*—the wood of the *nonu,* the stem— puts them together and bruises them and drinks. Then she will abort. *(Ko le fafine e tina'e ka vesia ki lona tina'e, ti 'au valu mai le tiale, o fakatasi mo le nonu 'akau o le nonu kuaga'i nonu o fa'i fakatasi, o palu, o inu, ti vilo lona tina'e.)*

12. *Uali (Mase samoana)*
(IP): The leaves are chewed and applied to wounds.

13. *Fau (Hibiscus tiliaceus;* Yellow hibiscus)
(IP) (ST): The shoots of this seaside shrub are used to make "relapse medicine" *(vai kita)*.

14. *'Afa (Neonauclea forsteri)*
(ST) (IP): The bark of this tree makes a potion given to a woman after childbirth.
 (IP): The woman whose stomach pains after giving birth. Not much blood has flowed down, so drink of that tree, and it will be well, her stomach will be well. *(Ko le fafine fānau ka e mamae lona manava. Lē'ai se lasi se ano mo le toto kiate ia, ti inu lēnā le la'akau, ti mālie 'oki lona manava.)*
 (ST): The trunk of the *'afa*, the base of the *nonu* and the *pua* are scraped by the woman who is pregnant and does not want her child; she drinks, then the child can fall. *(Ko le kuaga o le 'afa, ko le tafito o le nonu, ko le tafito o le pua, e valu mai e le fafine o ka e tina'e e sē fia ki lona toe, o inu, ti mafai ke vilo le toe.)*

15. *Kavakava-'atua (Piper vaupelii)*
(AP) (IP): The leaves of this handsome climbing plant are used to cool swellings and infection of the hands and feet (AP) and especially in the groin (IP). (ST) disputes the above and says that *kavakava-'atua* is used for ghost sickness *('āvaga)*.

16. *Valovalo (Premna taitensis)*
(ST) (IP) (AP): The leaves are used to make a liniment *(mili)* for babies who are feverish. It is also used for ghost sickness.

17. *Funavai (Tarenna sambucina)*
(ST) (IP) (AP): The leaves are used to make a potion/liniment for reducing filarial inflammations *(vai kulakula)*.

18. *Pua (Fagraea berteriana)*
(IP): It is used for stomach pains.
 (ST): An ingredient in an abortifacient (see under *'afa*).

19. *Koka (Bischofia javanica)*
(A) (IP) (ST): Scrapings from the trunk of this tree are used for mouth and throat infections.

20. *Talie (Terminalia catappus)*
(ST): The leaves are chewed and the juice dripped onto the lips of a baby whose mouth has been burned by hot food and drink.
 (IP) Drip it onto a wound to clot the blood *(ke malu le toto)*.

21. *Gatae (Erythrina variegata)*
(IP) (AP): The bark of the *gatae* is used to make a potion taken by women after childbirth *(le vai o le toka'ala)*.
 (IP): It is used by women who experience stomach pain after intercourse: "her

stomach and her back are painful because the man, her husband, is unwell, and he goes to her, his wife. After their 'sacrament' the wife's stomach is painful. Now come and scrape the *gatae*, fetch it, and drink it and recover." *(E mamae lona manava mo lona tu'a, e talie ko lona 'āvaga e masaki'ia. Ko le tagata, ko lona 'āvaga e masaki, ti 'au a ia kiate ia, ki lona 'āvaga. 'Oki lo laua sakalameta, ti mamae le manava o le fafine. Ti 'au valu mai le gatae. O 'au mai, o inu, ti mālie.)*

22. *Tiga'a-niu*, also called *Ti'a-niu (Phymatodes scolopendria)*
(ST): Chew fronds and mix with *koka (Bischofia javanica)* scrapings. Used for child with ulcerated mouth.
   (IP): Drops for the mouth.

23. *Tuitui (Aleurites moluccana;* Candlenut)
(MF) (ST): Scrapings from the bark are used for a child's sore throat.

24. *Mageo (Laportea interrupta)*
(ST): Scrapings from the trunk are used for treating ghost sickness. The leaves are used to treat painful swellings called *gugu*, which form on the joints (perhaps arthritic).
   (IP): *Mageo* is used in the same way as the *valovalo*, that is, as a liniment *(mili)* for young children who are sick.
   (MN): A potion for someone with swollen testicles, or rupture. The leaves, which sting like nettles, are pounded and the juice strained through a cloth and drunk.

25. *Vī-Papalagi (Psidium guava;* Yellow guava)
(ST): Potion for fatigue and body pain, made from the scrapings of the trunk.
   (PP, Yen): For diarrhoea.

26. *Kafika (Eugenia malaccensis;* Malay apple)
(ST): Chips of the bark are broken small, wrapped in cloth, and squeezed in water to extract juice. This infusion is drunk by children with cough.
   (IP): Potion made from the bark for bodily fatigue after strenuous work *(vai kita)*.
   (AP): For "relapse sickness" *(kita)* caused by returning to hard work before complete recovery.

27. *Ma'utofu (Urena lobata)*
(ST) (IP) (SL) (VS): Leaves from this shrub are crushed in the hand, then wrapped in a piece of cloth and steeped, rather perfunctorily, in a small amount of water to form what must be a very weak infusion, the greater part of which is drunk. The dregs *(su'a)* are used as a liniment *(mili)* to stroke the whole of the body in the gentle form of massage called *'amo'amo*. *Ma'utofu* is perhaps the best-known plant for making "relapse medicines" *(vai kita)*. As the plant also grows in New Caledonia, expatriate Futunans can continue its use there.
   One of the informants (IP) places great emphasis on administering the treatment after the onset of skin tenderness or internal pains which are regarded as

symptomatic for the types of *kita* called *kita kili* 'skin *kita*' and *kita kanofi* 'flesh *kita*'.

28. *Lau memei (Artoarpus communis;* Breadfruit leaves)
(ST) (IP): Leaf stalks are chewed and the juice dripped into an eye "that cannot see, and it will be well."

(ST): Scrapings from the trunk and other ingredients are mixed with coconut oil and made into a poultice to apply to injuries received from the spines of a fish.

29. *Pea,* also called *'Ukaki (Ocimum basilicum)*
(AP) (ST) (IP): Leaves make a lotion which is used to cool painful swellings, possibly filarial swelling.

30. *Sinu (Hoya australis)*
(IP): For stomach pains.

31. *Lau kofe (Bambusa sp.;* bamboo leaves)
(IP) (ST) (AP): Leaves are burned and the ash applied to burns.

32. *Seasea (Eugenia Corynocarpa)*
(AK) (ST) (IP): Leaves are chewed and applied as a liniment *(mili)* to painful swellings.

33. *Takafalu (Micromelum minitum)*
(AK) (ST): Leaves are used for filarial swelling *(masaki lasi),* either by chewing them (AK) or making a potion/liniment from them.

(IP): The *takafalu* is used to make drops *(tulu'i)* for headache.

34. *Lala (Vitex trifolia* and *Desmodium umbellatum)*
One of these species (it is not known which) is used for toothache (ST) (AK) (IP). According to (ST), orange leaves and *lala* leaves are chewed together and held against the sore tooth, which becomes very hot and the pain stops. The leaves, as is usually the case in Futunan medicine, should be taken in pairs *(soa).* In this case three pairs of orange leaves and three pairs of *lala* leaves are a good number.

35. *'U'ui (Derris trifoliata)*
This plant is often used as a fish poison (St. John and Smith 1971, 328); but in Futuna, according to (IP), the leaves are used to cool *(fakamomoko)* wounds.

36. *Aoa (Ficus prolixa;* banyan)
(AK): A lotion *(vai)* is made from its bark and applied to wounds.

37. *Salata (Nasturtium sarmentosum)*
(AK) (IP): The leaves are used to make headache drops *(tulu'i faa'ulu).*
(ST): A potion for sick children.

38. *Tona (Geophylla repens)*
(IP) (AK): This herb is used for mouth infections *(gutu papala).*

39. *Popo (Mussaenda raiatensis)*
(IP): The fruits are combined with five other (undetermined) ingredients to make a medicine to treat sick children.

40. *Soi (Dioscorea bulbifera;* yam sp.)
(AK) (IP): The young leaves are used as a dressing for infected wounds and sores.

41. *Ifi (Inocarpus edulis;* Tahitian chestnut)
(ST) (IP): Scrapings from the inner bark, mixed with *pilo,* according to (IP), are made into a potion/liniment which has many uses *(e maʻuke lona fai).*

(AK): The leaves are used to make eyedrops.

42. *Ago-ā-lulu (Zinziber zerumbet;* wild ginger)
(AK): A bright orange ointment is made from the root and used as a cosmetic and as protection against the sun.

(IP): Juice expressed from the leaves (?) is dripped onto wounds that are slow to heal.

43. *Malamea (Aglaia psilopetala)*
(IP): A potion is made from the bark and drunk by males suffering from swollen testicles.

44. *Poutea (Securinaga samoana)*
(ST) demonstrated the preparation of medicine for an ulcerated mouth as follows: the outer skin is shaved off *poutea* stem, and *mageo* stems are bent several times and pounded with a stone. Both are folded in a piece of cloth which is then dipped into water and squeezed so as to drip into the mouth. The taste is very mild.

(IP): A potion to treat spirit sickness *(ʻāvaga).*

(AK, Yen): Scrapings are used to make a potion for body pain.

45. *Tanetane-vao (Polyscias multijuga)*
(IP): It is used to make a potion for women who have stomach pains associated with intercourse *(e nofo mo lona ʻāvaga ka e mamae lona manava).*

46. *ʻUsi (Evodia hortensis)*
(AK): The leaves of this shrub are used to gently stroke *(mili)* swellings such as boils. Scrapings from the trunk make a potion for children's sore throat.

(IP): The strong-smelling leaves are used by women who practice medicine *(fafine fai faitoʻo)* to wash their patients. (Probably patients suffering from ghost sickness, as spirits dislike the strong smell.)

47. *Mapa (Diospyrus major)*
(AK): "Take the fruit, chew it, and spit it into the mouth of a child who has a sore throat."

7
Traditional Healing Practices of Rarotonga, Cook Islands
Josephine Baddeley

Rarotonga is the administrative center of the Cook Islands. In 1975, the time of this study, it had a population of approximately eight thousand. Rarotonga's first significant contact with Europeans was in the 1820s when the first missionaries settled there. From that time on, traders and settlers came to the island because of its fertile soils and cheap labor. In 1901 the Cook Islands were annexed by New Zealand, which continued to administer them until 1965, when they were accorded internal self-government. Throughout the period of its administration, New Zealand attempted to establish a central government and adequate health, welfare, and education services. The effect of these policies is most apparent today in Rarotonga, where public service is the largest employer. The impact of tourism is also readily apparent, and the life-style of most of the inhabitants has more in common with that of suburban New Zealand than a Polynesian peasantry.

Rarotonga has a well-established public health service, and the evident activity of nurses and western-trained doctors shows that Rarotongans readily utilize these facilities. In my first months of fieldwork I frequently saw people taken by ambulance to the hospital, and mothers assembling regularly at the village clinics to have their babies examined by the district nurse. It seemed that western medicine was readily appreciated by Rarotongans and, I assumed, had therefore largely supplanted any indigenous medical tradition. I soon became aware, however, that strange behavior, severe emotional stress, and some unusual physical handicaps were spoken of as illnesses—moreover, as illnesses of a particular type, *maki tūpāpaku* 'spirit illness'. It became clear that Rarotongans held ideas about such conditions that were not part of any western medical tradition.

Tūpāpaku, translated as "ghosts" or "spirits," had been described to me as beings generally encountered at night. They made disturbing

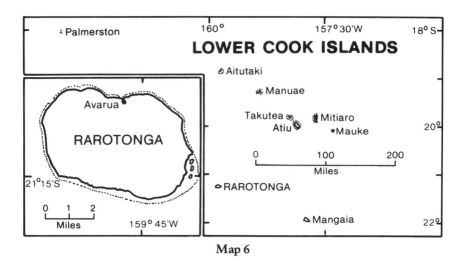

Map 6

noises and were particularly associated with *marae,* the traditional ceremonial courtyards. From this description I had assumed that Rarotongan *tūpāpaku* conformed to western ideas about ghosts. But the fact that they were associated with illness made me question my assumptions. To understand the connections between people, supernatural beings and illness, I had to examine the Rarotongan cosmology. The ideas related by my informants proved to be essential to an understanding of Rarotongan techniques of diagnosis and curing.

The analysis presented here derives from information obtained in interviews with recognized experts in traditional medicine as well as from casual conversations with many Rarotongans. Although I describe the various techniques of diagnosis and treatment which characterize traditional Rarotongan medicine, the main focus is on the ideas which support the medical tradition. In particular, I emphasize their ramifications for the treatment of "spirit sickness," a category of illness which Rarotongans do not believe to be recognized by western medicine.

IDEAS ABOUT THE SUPERNATURAL

In the Rarotongan conception of the universe there are three worlds, each with its own inhabitants who move between these worlds and communicate across them in various ways. People live in *ao nei* 'this world'. God, *vaerua* 'souls of the dead', angels, and saints live in *ao ra* 'that world'. The *aronga o te po* 'people of the *po*' live in the *po,* the "afterworld darkness or night." The *aronga o te po* are usually referred to as *tūpāpaku* 'spirits'.

God stays in "that world" and people stay in "this world" until they die and go to "that world" or the "afterworld." Spirits may move between "this world" and "that world." As well as moving between the worlds, the normal inhabitants of each may also communicate with one another in various ways. People send messages to God in their prayers and communicate with the spirits by making direct requests to them for help or with assistance of a *ta'unga* 'native healer', who acts as a spirit medium and communicates with spirits on their behalf. Spirits communicate with people in dreams and indicate their presence by unusual disturbances, particularly at night.

To many Europeans there appears to be a contradiction between the Rarotongans' apparently devout belief in Christianity and the recognition they give to the spirits of the dead. Rarotongans do not perceive this to be a contradiction. The Christian God is worshiped in church and the teachings of the pastor are accepted as important moral precepts for daily living. The pastor may also be appealed to in cases of illness. Biblical texts are the subject of lengthy intellectual discussion and are frequently quoted to emphasize a point of view. God is prayed to in the expectation that he will recognize and implement an individual's wishes. Since God is regarded as governing the cosmic order and determining the course of events in people's lives, he is asked to safeguard both communal undertakings and personal endeavors. But since spirits can intercede without a person's invitation and frequently do so in unpredictable ways, the spirits of one's close relatives are asked to intervene in personal dilemmas. Living people—in particular, healers—can manipulate the spirits, but this manipulation is not possible with the Christian God, to whom one may only make supplications.

SPIRITS AND HEALERS

Spirits are usually encountered at night, although they may also be present during the day. Spirits enter the world of the living from their graves, and people go to the grave of a deceased person when they wish to communicate with him. People often bury their relatives near their houses so that even after death they will remain close to one another. The secure and peaceful rest of the dead is ensured by burying them on their own land or in a place with which they were familiar, which also makes them less likely to trouble the living.

The moon is believed to influence the behavior of spirits, so that knowledge of the lunar calendar enables prediction of when spirits are likely to be most active. Spirits usually come at night in dreams or diguised as an animal or insect to warn, threaten, or simply converse with the living. When spirits assume the form of an animal or insect they are recognized by their unusual behavior. They can also take possession of a living person's body and communicate in this way. People I spoke with often mentioned being awakened at night by the feeling of a suffocating weight on their chest, which they attributed to being embraced by a spirit. The spirits communicate either directly or symbolically in dreams. When dreaming, people sometimes see dead relatives who have appeared to give them a message—perhaps to warn of a future event or simply to reassure them that they are content and are thinking of their kinsman. Spirits are also said to appear in dreams to tell people how to make medicines which will be effective for an illness they are trying to treat.

Many people look upon their deceased relatives as continuing to protect their interests. When they are in a distressing situation, they may appeal to their dead kinsmen for help, believing that they can exercise an influence on the affairs of the living. This benevolent influence is particularly felt on the family's land, where the spirits will frighten away trespassers. While spirits can help people in the ways mentioned, they demand respectful treatment in return and, if not treated appropriately, can exercise a malevolent influence on the living.

Some spirits maintain their contact with the living as spirit familiars of a native healer. There are two kinds of relationships between a healer and his familiar. In the first, a healer inherits a familiar which belongs to his family and has been passed down for generations from one healer to another. In the second, a familiar is sought by someone wishing to practice healing, and the familiar may in turn demand some form of compensation.

Spirit familiars usually appear when healers are in a trance or dreaming. Some healers summon their familiars at will while other familiars simply appear at significant times. When the healer is in a trance the spirit may take possession of his body; his voice changes. Often the healer himself has no recollection of what was said or what occurred during the trance.

A person cannot become a healer simply because of a wish to practice Maori medicine. He must be recognized by an established healer as having the dedication not only to learn the various techniques but to be available to patients at all hours of the day and night. Healers speak of their role as a special gift which imposes an obligation to use the gift for the benefit of others. The power of healing is considered to be reward enough in itself and healers are not allowed to accept any payment for their services. Although people sometimes return later with a present of food or clothing, the healer usually protests, saying that the services are not the sort that should be rewarded, lest the medicine lose its *mana* 'power'.

At the time of my study there were three healers practicing on Rarotonga who were well known to my informants: one elderly man, a young girl, and a middle-aged woman. None of them had wage employment and their standard of living was low by Rarotongan standards. People respected them for their knowledge and the help they gave to the sick, and were also afraid of the influence they had with the spirits. There were many others who had some of the skills of the well-known healers, but could not treat the wide variety of illnesses that the healers did. Thus, certain people were known to have the best remedies for particular complaints and they would be consulted by anyone suffering from those complaints. These people did not have a spirit familiar and had simply learned how to prepare certain medicines, either by experimenting or by learning from others.

IDEAS ABOUT ILLNESS

The Rarotongan word for illness is *maki*. There are two types of sickness which are distinguished from each other according to the causes to which they are attributed. Illnesses thought to be due to a natural cause are called *maki tikai* 'real sickness'; illnesses attributed to a supernatural agent are *maki tūpāpaku* 'spirit sickness'. *Maki māori* 'Maori sickness' is a term also used to refer to *maki tūpāpaku,* since people think of this kind of sickness as particularly characteristic of Maori people, even though Europeans sometimes fall sick with *maki tūpāpaku*.

To understand Rarotongan concepts of illness I conducted interviews with three practicing healers. One of them I observed for several weeks treating people in her home, and I discussed at length with her the type of therapy she used. Throughout the fourteen months of my fieldwork in Rarotonga, whenever people mentioned an illness they had suffered or spoke of other people's illness, I inquired about the treatment they had undergone and their own ideas about the causes of illness. Most people were happy to talk about these matters and often debated among themselves as to the causes of illness and the effectiveness of various treatments.

"Real illnesses" are illnesses which have only one cause. They are thought to be the direct consequences of certain events or actions of the sick person. People are said to catch colds or fevers from staying out in the rain or in cold weather without sufficient clothing, or to get stomach complaints from eating rotten food. "Spirit sicknesses," however, are attributed to more than one cause, since they are the result of the actions of both human and supernatural agents. Initially, a person might call upon the help of the spirits or provoke their intervention by some action which violates a *tapu* or offends them in some way. Informants say that unintentional misdemeanors do not necessarily result in a person's falling sick, but those who consciously break a *tapu* are likely to be punished by a spirit sickness. A person usually invokes the help of spirits to avenge an insult or harm he has suffered, often with unforeseen and disastrous consequences for the person who has given offense. Thus the primary cause of the spirit sickness is the action of a person which provokes the secondary cause, the intervention of the spirits, and this can be expressed in many different ways. To cure a spirit sickness, both the primary and secondary causes must be recognized and treated appropriately.

THE CLASSIFICATION OF ILLNESS

In an attempt to determine some of the ways in which Rarotongans conceptualize illness, I asked a number of informants to classify a list of ninety illnesses into similar groups. (It was irrelevant to this classification whether an illness was caused by a supernatural agent or not; informants were simply asked to group similar illnesses together.) I used terms collected from Savage (1962) and MacKenzie (1973) and then checked these terms against my own informants' descriptions of the various illnesses. This cross-check revealed that there was some difference of opinion concerning both the symptoms which these terms described and appropriate treatment. Informants also attributed illnesses to different causes and differed in the accounts they gave of the sequence of stages through which an illness progressed.

Although there was a considerable divergence of opinion in the way informants classified illnesses, a few basic principles did emerge. People classified illnesses according to the region of the body affected and also according to the sequence of events. Thus they grouped together measles, chicken pox, boils, and swellings as all being skin conditions.

There was also a particular category of illness termed 'ira. 'Ira is translated by Savage as "a mark such as a birthmark; a mole or moles; freckles or other natural marks on the skin" (1962, 74). Although their descriptions agreed with Savage's definition, informants said that 'ira most commonly was a type of illness contracted by babies and that it took various forms: 'ira moe—the child sleeps much longer than usual and may wake up showing only the whites of his eyes; 'ira uti—when teething starts the baby gets convulsions; 'ira miti—a bumpy skin rash; 'ira i'i matangi—a red rash on the face.

Informants often referred to an illness as *vera* 'hot' or *anu* 'cold', and they said that if an illness for which a "hot" medicine is appropriate was treated with a "cold" one, or vice versa, the result could be fatal. Although both illnesses and medicines were classified as hot or cold, not all medicines or illnesses were so classified. From the informants' descriptions, it seemed that the hot or cold designation refers to the temperature of the sick person's body or the affected area of the body.

These preliminary investigations did not reveal any comprehensive classificatory scheme. Rather, it seems that there is a wide divergence of opinion concerning both illness classification and diagnosis.

DIAGNOSIS

Those initially involved in diagnosing an illness are the sick person and members of his family and household. They decide whether or not the illness is serious enough to warrant consulting a healer or any other medical expert. If they decide that the illness is one for which they have a remedy, they will use their own homemade medicine. If expert advice is sought, the source of that advice will depend on the nature of the illness and also the familiarity of those making the initial diagnosis with the various types of treatment. Families who have been in New Zealand for a long time, or who do not have ready access to a practicing healer, will usually consult the western-trained doctor at the hospital. Others who have a healer in the family, or are accustomed to seeking a healer's advice, will consult the healer. If the healer's treatment or the doctor's medicine does not remove all the symptoms, then an alternative form of treatment may be attempted.

I was told by one woman that she had been suffering from stomach pains which were becoming increasingly severe, and as the doctor could not identify the complaint, he sent her home with some pain suppressants. The pain intensified instead, so her aunt took her to a healer, who massaged her stomach. After the massage the pain became unbearable. Her mother, fearing that she might die, then took her to the hospital. The doctor recognized an acute appendicitis and operated immediately. The massage had merely aggravated the condition.

The Rarotongan attitude to treatment is essentially pragmatic and eclectic. People will try a treatment recommended by friends even while undergoing a different course of treatment. It is not thought that an illness can be cured by only one type of treatment, and what is effective for one person might be ineffective for another. The treatment of illness is a process of experimentation, and people are generally very open to trying several different cures, both European and Maori. Many Rarotongans, however, did express a fear of surgical operations, which have no equivalent in Maori medicine.

The greater frequency with which people consult European rather than Maori experts is a reflection of their growing familiarity with European medicine and a decline in the number of practicing healers. Yet the increasing acceptance of western medicine does not seem to have affected the traditional explanation of certain illnesses as being caused by spirits.

Diagnosis proceeds along with treatment and changes according to the person's response to the medicine given him. Informants told me that if a person tries too many medicines he will become very sick. It is accepted that European methods are superior for treating illnesses such as appendicitis or pneumonia whereas Maori medicines are used, at least initially, for minor complaints and for those which are diagnosed as "spirit sickness."

MAORI MEDICINES

Vairākau Maori 'Maori medicines' consist, for the most part, of natural ingredients, as one would expect from the words *vai* 'water' and *rākau* 'plant'. They are used in the treatment of both "real sickness" and "spirit sickness." It is not only the natural properties of the ingredients which affect the cure, but also the influence that supernatural beings may have on the curing process. Throughout all stages, from the initial formulation in the mind of the healer to the collection of ingredients and their preparation and administration to the sick person, any medicine may be rendered more, or less, effective by the intervention of supernatural powers.

Every informant, even children, knew a few cures for common ailments such as insect bites. The best-known medicines are the *vairākau mimi* 'diuretics' and *vairākau 'aka'eke* 'laxatives'. The reason people give for using these medicines is to rid the body of impurities. It is held that many illnesses, such as asthma and certain skin complaints, are the result of "bad feces" stored in the body and should be treated with laxatives. Informants say that diuretics are easy to prepare and their effect can be easily seen. They are used to treat venereal disease, hepatitis, styes of the eye, and skin diseases.

Just as there is a distinction between hot and cold illnesses, there is also a distinction between hot and cold medicines. All medicines labeled hot are heated, while those labeled cold are not. One informant said that certain plants have cold properties—for example, the leaves of the hibiscus and *cordyline terminalis*. Cold medicines are said to work by taking the heat out of the illness. Informants could not state the specific properties of a medicine which caused it to be labeled hot or cold. They were adamant, however, that hot illnesses should always be treated with cold medicines and that these medicines should have no contact with red materials, which they say have hot properties. Similarly, cold illnesses should always be treated with hot medicines.

Ingredients

The basic ingredients of Maori medicine are plants, most of which are considered weeds and are found in the wild bush. The great variety of ingredients causes some people to refer to the taking of medicine as *kai tutae* 'eating feces'. The emphasis on natural ingredients is such that it will often be stipulated that the water used is to be taken from streams, not tap water. Another pure liquid used is the juice from drinking coconuts. It is also undesirable to use plants which have been sprayed with an insecticide.

The most common method of preparing medicines is to pound the plant material in a wooden bowl, collect it in a cloth and wring the juice from the crushed leaves. The juice may then be sweetened by the addition of sugarcane juice, added to water and drunk, or inhaled or applied to an injury. A common method of treating certain illnesses is to make a steam bath by placing hot rocks in water. The patients stands or sits over the bath and is covered with blankets so that no heat escapes.

Rules Governing the Use of Medicines

Medicines are rendered effective by virtue of the *mana* 'power' of supernatural beings. In the Rarotongan view, these beings may be the Christian God, the spirits of dead relatives, or the spirit familiar of the healer. Many healers who receive their recipes for medicines from a familiar still conceive of the ingredients as having been created by God, and they will pray for his help before making the medicine. Some healers also use the Bible as an aid to treatment. A text is selected by the healer, who is guided in his choice by God, and given to the sick person to memorize so as to put him in the right frame of mind to render the cure effective. Some medicines are affected by the supernatural to a greater degree than others. Some medicines have great *mana* and are often attended by rigid proscriptions. These medicines are of two types: those which are revealed to a healer in a dream, and those which belong to a particular family and can be used only by members of that family. In some cases these medicines cannot be revealed to others without losing their power.

Medicines may have a power of their own which affects people whether they are taking them or not. I was told by a healer that she had cured a person by removing some old Maori medicine from her house. When people are being treated with these particularly powerful medicines they are thought to be in a *tapu* state and must observe certain restrictions, such as not taking any kind of European medicine during the course of treatment. The power of some medicines also affects any waste material left after their preparation, and this material must be carefully disposed of.

Medicines are affected by the phases of the moon. I was told that medicines for children are most likely to be affected by the phases of the moon. There are three principal times in the lunar month when children should take medicine: at new moon, at full moon, and during the first night of the last quarter. In addition, medicines given by the spirits often have to be taken at certain times of the month to make them effective.

Medicines can be affected by the weather. Certain medicines are not effective on cold days; laxatives, for example, will not work on cold days because the sick person's body will not loosen up. On hot days very cold medicines are warmed first before being taken. In addition to the weather and the lunar cycle, medicines can also be affected by daily changes such as the rise and fall of the tide and the time of the day.

When the medicine is being prepared there may be certain signs which indicate to the healer that the medicine will not be effective. The following signs tell the healer that spirits are trying to affect the medicine: (1) if the leaves of the plant the healer has chosen for the medicine are dead when he comes to pick them, or if the plant material changes color after it has been ground up; (2) if an insect alights on the plant being used while the healer is gathering the leaves. (The insect may be a form taken by the spirit who does not want the sick person to be cured.) If the healer originally thought that he was dealing with a "real sickness," these signs would indicate that it is in fact a "spirit sickness." Sometimes the healer will then abandon the treatment, or he might continue it to give the person some hope of recovery.

Massage

Massage is a form of treatment often used instead of, or in conjuction with, herbal medicines. A wide variety of "real sickness" is treated by massage—influenza, strained muscles, headaches, strokes, and fever—as is "spirit sickness." Many people know how to give simple massage to relieve muscular pain, but few individuals specialize in massage. At the time of my study, a seventy-year-old man in Rarotonga was still occasionally giving massages for which he was an acknowledged expert. Interviews were conducted with this masseur, who demonstrated his techniques. He maintained that he had never failed to cure a person unless they had come when the illness was already too far advanced.

The masseur first asks the sick person the history of his illness and then seats him on a small stool with his back to the masseur. Sometimes the masseur uses a patent rubifacient (e.g. Vicks Vaporub), or coconut oil. The masseur recognizes that there are certain important pressure points in the body, and generally the part of the body massaged is not the painful area, to avoid aggravating the damage. The masseur uses long stroking movements and applies pressure with his thumbs. The reason he gave for massage being an effective treatment was that it caused the blood to circulate. He said that when people sit around and take insufficient exercise, their blood becomes stagnant and this causes the person to become ill.

The masseur told me that he had also cured people suffering from spirit sickness. He said that it was easy to tell when people were suffering from spirit sickness because of their bizarre behavior and their attempts to avoid being treated. At the beginning of such a massage the masseur attempts to discover with his hands where the spirit is hiding in the person's body. When possessed by a spirit the patient might undergo violent convulsions; it then becomes necessary for an assistant to hold him down while the treatment proceeds. Massage by itself is not usually sufficient to cure a spirit sickness and often the masseur has to find out which spirit is causing the illness. If, by consultation with the person, the masseur discovers the identity of the spirit, he may be able to shame the spirit into leaving by calling out its name and telling it to leave the person.

Massage is not a method which is employed exclusively. It is usually practiced in conjuction with herbal treatments to cure some of the physical manifestations of the illness, or with the help of spirit mediums to treat spirit sickness.

THE TREATMENT OF SPIRIT SICKNESS

When a sick person comes to see a healer, the healer asks about the history of the illness so that information can be gained from the account of the symptoms. His main concern is to discover whether or not the illness is a spirit sickness and how the sickness was caused. Usually the healer is not concerned with the immediate circumstances in which the illness began, but rather with the significant events preceding its onset. The consultation proceeds by the healer talking to the person to discover what stresses or troubles he might have been experiencing. If he is aware of having offended someone, or of having been in a distressing situation and appealing to the spirits for help, this might suggest a possible reason for the illness. The healer does not automatically accept the person's explanation, however, and relies instead on the advice received from his familiar.

During the consultation the healer carefully observes the sick person's behavior since certain symptoms may indicate a spirit sickness. Such indications include the following:

1. A person possessed by a spirit might cover himself with blankets, swear at the healer, and try to prevent treatment. This reaction is said to be that of the spirit, who does not want to be driven from the body. A person who is possessed may also hold his hands tightly together or mislead the healer about the location of the pain in his body.
2. If one of the symptoms of the illness is a muscular pain which does

not remain in one place but shoots around the body, it is probably a spirit sickness.
3. Spirit sickness sometimes has its onset at sunset, becoming progressively worse during the night, and is most powerful around midnight when the spirits are most influential.
4. Psychological disturbance may be considered a spirit sickness. People are said to become crazy if they devote themselves fanatically to a cause or a person. Mental illness can be the result of a broken heart. Too much studying or mental effort also produce this type of illness. The healer must determine whether or not a particular case is a spirit sickness, and it is said that a mental illness is easier to cure if it is caused by spirits than it is if it is a "real sickness."

After the initial consultation with the sick person, the healer usually attempts to contact his familiar. (Some ask the sick person to pray with them for the success of the treatment.) The healer sometimes communicates with his familiar in a trancelike state; at other times he might use additional aids such as playing cards. The healer I observed using playing cards assigned attributes to the cards which represented important influences in the person's life. The juxtaposition of the cards as they were dealt onto the table told the healer what emotions were affecting the various significant actors in the person's life and what significant events might have occured. After studying the cards for some time, the healer told the sick person what each card represented and how they were affecting him. The person then affirmed the interpretation and gave additional information about the people and events which might have been the cause of the illness.

Not all treatment sessions involve the same degree of consultation between sick person and healer, since some healers do not need help in determining the diagnosis. They say that they have all the information revealed to them by their spirit familiar even before the person has arrived for consultation. The familiar will have described the sick person, the symptoms of his illness, and may even have given the remedy for it.

The discussion between the healer and sick person often has the effect of unburdening him of guilt he has been carrying for some wrongdoing. Once the healer has confronted the person with his misdeed, he will often admit his guilt and apologize to the person he had offended, if this is what the healer has asked him to do. The confession then has a remarkable effect on the sick person's psychological well-being. The acknowledgement of transgression is thus part of the cure, and if the sick person refuses to acknowledge his fault, he cannot expect to be cured. The healer cannot force the person to take the steps he considers appropriate, but usually his diagnosis becomes known and when this is endorsed by public opinion the person will usually follow the healer's advice. Once the offended party (which may be a person or a spirit) has been appeased, the most important part of the cure has been effected. The healer might make some medicine for the sick person, in addition, but this is not regarded as a vital part of the treatment.

A person who is possessed by a spirit is sometimes given a hot bath in which the leaves of a fern have been crushed. Spirits are said to dislike these leaves. Much of the treatment for possession, in addition to the massage mentioned before, involves the healer's talking to the spirit. Often the healer can shame the spirit and make it leave the person's body, but the healer must be careful not to make the spirit angry or violent, as this might cause the person's death.

Although there is no explicit Rarotongan classification of the causes of spirit sickness, a healer I talked with offered the following principles.

(1) The sick person might have caused his own illness when in stress by appealing to a spirit for help, usually a close relative. This request makes the person vulnerable to the power of the spirit, who might even attempt to remove him from the unpleasant situation by making him become ill and die. Those who mourn too deeply for their dead kin are likely to succumb to spirit sickness in this way because the spirit of the dead person may try to take the mourner with it into death. People are thus warned against becoming too emotionally involved with another person. I was told that a woman from the Outer Islands had come to a healer in Rarotonga because since her arrival there she had become seriously ill and her condition was deteriorating. Her husband had not wanted her to leave, had given her no money for the trip, and was neglecting their children in her absence. The healer discovered, through her cards, that this situation had caused the woman to appeal to her dead grandmother who had looked after her when she was young. Thus her illness was caused by the grandmother's attempts to remove her from her distress. The healer advised her that the only way she would get well was by ceasing to appeal to her grandmother and wishing to be taken away from her troubles.

(2) A person might become ill as a result of being cursed by someone whom they have offended or disobeyed. Healers, titleholders, and pastors are thought to have special *mana* which makes their curses particularly powerful, so care must be taken not to offend them. In addition, everyone is vulnerable to the curses of certain close relatives, especially parents. I was told of one case when a man came to consult the healer about his son who was ill and behaving strangely. The boy had been studying hard and reading a lot. His mother did not want him to continue at school and tried to make him get a job. At this he left home, which further infuriated his mother, and then became seriously ill. The healer

talked to the boy and discovered that his sickness had been caused by his mother's curse. The boy would be cured only if the mother revoked her curse.

Some people are said to practice a certain type of cursing known as *kai tangata,* literally "eating people." I was told of one old woman who had been ill, taken to hospital, and placed in a ward with others much younger than herself. She was not expected to live for very long, but she survived while others in the same ward died. It was said that she had bargained with the spirits to take the lives of the other patients instead of hers.

(3) Whereas the last-mentioned type of spirit sickness involves a person who deliberately curses another, people can also unconsciously cause others to become ill. If a person has been gravely insulted or annoyed by another, his displeasure may provoke a reaction from a spirit who looks after his interests. The spirit avenges the insulted party by causing the person who offended him to become sick.

One such case involved a man whose brother-in-law had planted banana trees in a place where he had been asked not to. The brother-in-law became paralyzed and was unable to walk. After spending some time in hospital, where he received no effective treatment, he consulted a healer. The healer called a meeting of the sick person's family to discuss the illness and uncover any dissension in the family. The sick man's wife told the assembled family that she had seen an old woman wandering around their house, and when she described the woman they realized that it was the spirit of her dead grandmother. The healer said that this spirit must be intervening on behalf of the sick man's brother-in-law, who admitted that he still bore a grudge about the bananas. The healer then said the sick person could only be cured if he was nursed by his brother-in-law, to demonstrate to the grandmother's spirit that there was no longer any ill-feeling between them. This was done and the man recovered.

(4) A person can become sick as punishment for another who is closely related to the sick person. In these cases it is usually children who become sick as a result of their parents' transgressions. Rarotongans refer to the biblical quotation "the sins of the fathers are visited on the sons" as an explanation for the spirit sicknesses which are caused in this way.

One woman told me the story of her young baby's illness. She took him to the hospital and the doctor could not do anything for him, so she took him to a healer, against her husband's wishes as he did not believe in the healer's power. The healer said that the child had been made ill because of the parents' frequent arguments, which had provoked the wife's dead grandmother to intervene by making the child sick as a way of punishing the husband. The healer said the child would get well if they were reconciled and thereby ceased angering the grandmother.

Another kind of case is that of children who become sick when given the wrong name. A person's name must be chosen with care because some names are the property of families and cannot be given to those who have no right to them. Naming a child gives the person who bestows the name certain rights over the child, so it is not a privilege to be used casually. It is said that ancestral spirits can be offended by the wrong choice of name, and will demonstrate their displeasure by making the child sick so as to punish those who have named the child wrongly. The child will get well once the name is changed.

CONCLUSION

Rarotongans acknowledge that western medical techniques are superior for the treatment of many readily diagnosed conditions. It is for the treatment of psychosomatic illness that they prefer traditional healers. It is obvious that the efficacy of healers in this area is due to their thorough appreciation of the sources of stress in Rarotongan society, and their ability to elicit from the sick person the cause of this stress and then eliminate it.

The possibility of incurring a spirit sickness acts as a deterrent to socially undesirable behavior. Rather than forcibly preventing someone from carrying out their intentions, the Rarotongan way is simply to point out the probable consequences of undesirable actions. Actions and attitudes which are said to incur spirit sickness thus indicate a code of conduct which is particularly applicable to relations between kinsmen. The judicial code founded on New Zealand's legal system does not regard as reprehensible much of the behavior traditionally considered immoral from the standpoint of the expectations and obligations entailed in kin relationships. It is in these relationships that the influence of spirits is most apparent. In the Rarotongan view spirit sickness, although having physical symptoms, is more involved with a breakdown in social relations than it is with physiology.

Healers therefore spend a good deal of time in consultation with the sick person and his family. These consultations are not affected by considerations of time and payment. People are encouraged to air any grievances which might be causing tension and stress within the family. The sick person is not treated as an isolate, but rather is considered in the context of family relationships.

It is important that western doctors understand this concept of illness and the sources of stress; Rarotongans consider it as much a part of their medical tradition as everyday minor complaints. Such an understanding would go a long way toward improving doctor-patient relationships by enhancing appreciation of situations which are not at all bizarre or eccentric in the context of traditional Rarotongan medicine.

8
Physical and Social Boundaries in Pukapukan Theories of Disease
Julia A. Hecht

This chapter considers the significance of physical and social boundaries in Pukapukan ideas about the causes of disease.[1] While Pukapukans appear to have a fairly low level of anxiety about contamination and purity, the maintenance of certain boundaries is important and the crossing of these boundaries figures prominently in explanations of the occurrence of illness. Earlier studies have described the importance of the physical boundaries of the island in Pukapukan social organization (Hecht 1976; 1977; 1981). These boundaries are also important in Pukapukan theories of disease. Ideas about "boat sickness," gods who deliver disease or deny protection from it, and ancestral spirits who inflict disease on misbehaving descendants all find a rationale in Pukapukan beliefs about their island world and its relation to other places and peoples.

AN ATOLL PERSPECTIVE

Pukapuka is a coral atoll located approximately 1144 km northwest of Rarotonga, the administrative center of the Cook Islands. The atoll is comprised of three islets with a total land area of about 607 hectares. Pukapuka's closest neighbors are Nassau Island, 67 km to the southeast, also inhabited by Pukapukans (Vayda 1958); Manihiki and Rakahanga, over 320 km to the northwest; and American Samoa, nearly 640 km to the southwest.

The atoll's history expresses the theme of isolation. Pukapukan history holds that the first Pukapukan sprang from the "rock" of the atoll itself; the "head of the rock" *(te ulu o te watu)* is the atoll's traditional name. A visiting god told the Pukapukan man to find a wife on another island; he did so and returned to the atoll (Beaglehole and Beaglehole 1938, 375–

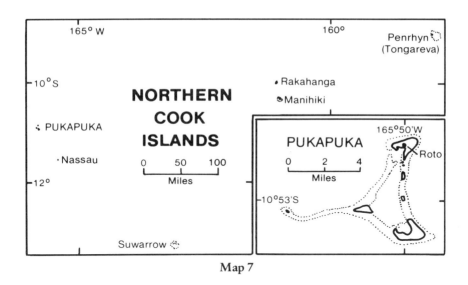

Map 7

77). The major chiefly line, and subsequently the rest of the Pukapukan people, descend from this couple.

Between that legendary past and the mid-nineteenth century, only two female survivors of a drift voyage from Manihiki are thought to have settled permanently on the atoll and to have left descendants (Beaglehole and Beaglehole 1938, 393–94). Although the indigenous history tells of sporadic voyaging and occasional visitors to the atoll, there was no regular interchange before missionization in 1857. The island has remained relatively isolated and self-sufficient to the present time; usually no more than three boats arrive at Pukapuka during a year.

While Pukapukans have been aware of the outside world from the moment of their genesis from their own land under the gaze of the visiting god, they view their atoll as somewhat of a last outpost. For example, the Pukapukan story of the division of coconuts among the Polynesian peoples holds that Pukapuka was almost forgotten and, when finally remembered, received only a tiny, wizened nut as the seed from which its stock grows (Beaglehole and Beaglehole 1938, 82).

The island attitude is typified by a self-conscious pride which is more accepting of outsiders (who rarely stay long in any case) than of innovations, which are accepted only cautiously (Beckett 1964). Even outsiders were challenged by island guards before they were allowed to pass the boundaries of the atoll (Beaglehole and Beaglehole 1938, 374).

In addition to the outside world, the distant lands beyond the reef, there is the *po*, an underworld or afterworld believed to be entered through a hole in the reef itself (Beaglehole and Beaglehole 1938, 327).

The *po* is inhabited by gods and the spirits of the ancestral dead and is also accessible to the living in dream or trance. Spirit beings from both of these other lands, the land beyond the reef and the underworld of the *po*, figure prominently in the causation and treatment of disease.

OUTSIDE CONTACT AND DISEASE: SOME EARLY HISTORY

When European explorers first visited the islands of Polynesia, the populations they encountered were probably fairly healthy aside from some endemic conditions. But the explorers brought new disease agents and new modes of clothing and housing which soon altered the receptivity of the Polynesian hosts.

For Pukapuka, effective contact and the beginnings of more or less regularly recorded history began with the arrival of London Missionary Society teachers from the Lower Cook Group in 1857. The presence of mission teachers entailed the periodic visit of missionary visitors, who wrote of island mores and events in their journals and letters.

The first population estimate was 750 in 1862 (Gill 1862). Shortly thereafter, in 1863, blackbirders took away about 140 Pukapukans for labor in Peru. Only two at most ever returned and this episode does not appear to have been associated with the drastic depopulation due to disease that occurred in other islands (Maude 1981).

Chalmers reported in 1870 that the Pukapukans "did not look so well as the natives to Eastward" (presumably those of Manihiki and Rakahanga) and estimated the population at five hundred (Chalmers 1870). After an epidemic of an unrecorded nature late in 1871, the population was reported to be down to three hundred persons (Vivian 1871–72), although this estimate may be unreasonably low (McArthur 1967).

Some of the ill health may have been derived from the return of a small group engaged to do plantation labor and domestic service in Hawaii. Apparently about twenty returned to Pukapuka in 1869 and they brought leprosy back with them (Beaglehole and Beaglehole 1938, 5).

The scattered reports of this leprosy are curious. By 1877 William Wyatt Gill reported that the "terrible leprosy introduced seven years ago from the Sandwich Islands has nearly died out, only four cases remaining" (Gill 1877). And in 1879, he recorded that it had disappeared and that in fact he "saw no skin disease whatever; no scrofula. Elephantiasis and its kindred complaints are however common" (Gill 1879).[2]

In 1909, however, a Dr. Gartley found two lepers and reported "something obscure in the occurrence of these cases of leprosy in this remote and little-visited island, for the people assert that they had no previous cases of this disease, and that the two men have never been away from the island" (Gudgeon 1909). Perhaps this was a conscious denial of a dread disease, for the Pukapukans had adopted the Christian Bible enthusiastically by this time. It is also possible, however, that the leprosy following 1869 and that of 1909 were classified as different diseases by the Pukapukans.

While Dr. Gartley may have introduced the idea of outside contact in his questions about the source of the leprosy, the recognition of outside sources of disease is also a crucial part of the indigenous etiology. Even if there was a common source for both outbreaks, the chain of transmission from 1869 to 1909 was long enough so that while those in 1869 were recognized as having a disease from outside, those in 1909 might have been considered to have an indigenous affliction. Indigenous categories corresponding to this distinction between "outside" and "inside" will be discussed below in relation to causes of disease.

THE PUKAPUKAN PEOPLE TODAY

Although Pukapuka itself has remained relatively isolated, Pukapukans have traveled in increasingly greater numbers during the decades since World War II. Today they are far more widespread than ever before.

Pukapukans began to settle in Rarotonga after a tidal wave in Pukapuka in 1914 (Beaglehole and Beaglehole 1938, 12). When I was there in the early 1970s, Pukapukans seemed to regard Rarotonga primarily as a way station from which they would either return to Pukapuka or proceed on to New Zealand. Few Pukapukans have claims to land in Rarotonga and they are regarded there as a physically and linguistically distinct outgroup.

The first Pukapukan to settle in New Zealand arrived after World War I, but movement in that direction did not begin in earnest until the late 1950s (Beckett 1964) and developed more intensely in the later 1960s and early 1970s. While there were 7 men and 4 women in New Zealand in 1951, a community count in 1963 put the Pukapukan population at 138, including 53 men, 33 women, and 52 children. In 1974, except for the 735 Pukapukans on the atoll itself, there were more Pukapukans in Auckland, New Zealand, than in all other places combined. Much of the Auckland community appears to be permanently settled there. From the approximately 600 Pukapukans in Auckland in 1976, a sample of 170 employed persons showed that most are blue-collar laborers. About 54 percent of the Pukapukan women in New Zealand were employed in 1976 (Hecht 1978).

Of 295 Pukapukans age twenty or more, resident in Pukapuka in 1974, 243 (82.4 percent) had visited Rarotonga and 32 (10.8 percent) had visited New Zealand at some point in their lives. The average length of stay in both Rarotonga and New Zealand was 3.9 years (Hecht 1978).

Through travel and the presence of some Europeans and medical personnel as well as other Cook Islanders on the atoll over the years, Pukapukans have been exposed to western medical ideas and practices and to other Polynesian ideas and techniques. In the rest of this chapter, I will describe some traditional Pukapukan theories of disease and changes they have undergone. The available data enable only a preliminary sketch of what is surely a very complex set of phenomena.

CAUSES OF DISEASE

The traditional etiology of disease involved three categories: the first focused on the intervention of a god, the second centered on the revenge of an ancestral spirit, and the third involved foreign spirits in the incidence of epidemic disease (Beaglehole and Beaglehole 1938, 335ff.).

The Beagleholes present a scenario for disease brought by the intervention of a god. If a man is injured either physically or mentally by another and wants revenge, he consults a god of his lineage. For a minor injury and a simple revenge, the god may be consulted anywhere by the injured party. If the injury and requisite revenge are serious, a priest must intercede with the god. If the god decides to act, he or an attendant spirit will insert a disease object into the body of the offender, through the mouth or the anus. This object causes sickness by twisting up, gnawing at, or sticking into vital organs.

> [The offender] now falls sick, and calls into consultation a medicine man, who, after a digital exploration of the parts affected, diagnoses the trouble. The medicine man consults the god of his lineage, and procures instructions for removing the foreign body from the patient. With his fingers he squeezes the patient's body and draws out the foreign object. He keeps his hand closed, lest the object try to escape back into the body, but the patient's relatives gather round and feel the hand of the medicine man so as to be assured that the object is really inside it. Then he crushes the disease object and throws it into the fire, so killing the spirit that entered into the object within the patient . . . [who] should now get well. (Beaglehole and Beaglehole 1938, 336)

From my observations in Pukapuka, it appeared that digital diagnosis and deep pressure massage are still the primary modes of diagnosis and treatment. In the early 1970s, however, I did not hear of disease being attributed to intervention by traditional gods. All Pukapukans are adherents of either the Cook Islands Christian Church, Roman Catholic Church, or the Seventh Day Adventist faith, and those elements of traditional religious belief that remain are not easily shared with outsiders.

The second category of disease, that caused by malicious spirits of the dead, is also illustrated by the Beagleholes (1938, 337). They tell the story of a man named Yawani from Tongareva or Penrhyn, the northernmost of the Cook Islands, who lived in Pukapuka in the mid-1800s just after the arrival of the first mission teachers. The pastor insulted Yawani, who died soon afterward from an injury suffered by falling from a tree. Yawani's soul wandered the island and appeared to cause the pastor's wife to fall ill. Levi, or Luavavai, a famous Pukapukan seer and healer, sought the *aitu* or spirit:

> Levi performed the pigeon *(lupe)* ritual and called on his gods to help him wrestle with the spirit. . . . Levi's gods had rallied to his aid. The gods surrounded the *aitu* so it could not escape; Levi rushed at it with a stick and struck it several times. Some blood fell on the ground (and teeth and a head as well, say some!), and this was taken as a token that Levi had killed the spirit. Further proof was that the pastor's wife got well and the soul was never seen again. (Beaglehole and Beaglehole 1938, 337)

Vindictive spirits of the dead were cited several times as causes of disease while I was in Pukapuka. In particular, the sickness and death of a twenty-three-year-old woman was attributed to her maternal grandmother, whose deathbed request the woman or her mother had apparently ignored. The social pressure on survivors to obey these requests is strong, and ignoring a request is a plausible reason for retribution from the afterworld.

I have no information on the early visits of this young woman to indigenous practitioners before she saw the Cook Islands medical practitioner. The lay opinion, however, particularly of the adolescents, was that hers was some kind of sexually transmitted disease, as could be seen in the swelling of her abdomen that had initially suggested pregnancy. A large tumor was successfully removed some months before her death.

Spirits of the sick, as well as those of the dead, are feared. Dreaming of the woman during her final illness was held to be a bad omen. As she became increasingly weak, people were afraid of her ghost both during the day and at night. Although ghosts may roam anywhere, the kin group graveyards are especially to be avoided at night. Pukapukans are perfectly comfortable in these areas during the daylight hours.

Many cases of family disability, including congenital deformities, apparent susceptibility to filiarial swelling, and deafness, are attributed to behavioral lapses, such as theft or incest in previous generations, which gods or ancestors punish by visiting disease upon succeeding generations. I will discuss this belief further under the rubric of susceptibility to disease.

The third traditional category of illness involved the spirits of foreign dead or foreign gods who either visited the island on their own or came with visiting voyagers or a drift canoe. These foreign spirits and gods specialized in epidemic sickness (Beaglehole and Beaglehole 1938, 337).

While I did not hear it cast in terms of superhuman spirits, the attribution of illness to outside contact is still pervasive. For Pukapukans on the island itself, the major type of disease which corresponds to this third category is "boat sickness" *(te maki payi)*. Prior et al. (1966, 32) discuss the phenomenon under the heading "Non-Tuberculous Chest Conditions":

> Intercurrent upper and lower respiratory infections are uncommon on Pukapuka, but occur with normal frequency in Rarotonga.
>
> The way in which an acute viral respiratory infection can spread through an isolated community was shown very clearly on Pukapuka. Introduced by passengers on the boat, it quickly spread through the community and it is estimated that around 85% of the entire community were affected to varying extent. . . . The condition is called by the Pukapukans "the sickness and cough of the boat" and is a well-recognized phenomenon.

Boat sickness was a continuing concern during my stay in 1972–74. Mumps, for example, was delivered to the atoll on the boat arriving on August 9, 1972. There were sixty active cases on October 9, two months later. On February 12, 1973, about six months after the initial case, there was at least one active case remaining. There may have been further cases of which I was not aware; no deaths resulted.

It is not clear whether cases of boat sickness today are regarded as natural and biological or as supernatural. Traditionally, this third category of disease was considered particularly malevolent and difficult to control, requiring not just treatment of the patients but killing the foreign spirit itself which was abroad somewhere on the atoll (Beaglehole and Beaglehole 1938, 337).

While epidemic disease was especially associated with foreign spirits, in one sense all three traditional categories linked disease with superhuman agency from *outside* the ordinary island world, from either the underworld of Pukapukan gods and spirits or the non-Pukapukan world. But disease was not simply associated with physical boundaries; moral boundaries were also important. One became sick because of a lapse in one's own or a relative's behavior. This was true even in the case of disease inflicted by a foreign spirit or god; had it not been for a lapse in rectitude of some sort one's own god would have offered protection sufficient to counter the foreign malevolence.

SUSCEPTIBILITY TO DISEASE

While physical boundaries divided Pukapukans from the outside and underworld, where bearers of disease originate, the observance of moral boundaries on the island was insurance against the occurrence of disease. Ultimately, someone's misbehavior—an omission or commission—was responsible for disease. Accordingly, when the cause could not be found and treatment did not avail, it was customary to hold a confessional over the patient to determine an appropriate course of action (Beaglehole and Beaglehole 1938, 338). This aspect of confessional still seems to be part of the social character and attraction of the sickbed.

Particularly important social boundaries concern sexuality and property relations. While Pukapukans have a realistic attitude toward sexual behavior generally, it is expected to occur within certain limits. First, sex is private, and under ordinary circumstances it should be engaged in only in a secluded place away from other people (Vayda 1961). Disease can be transmitted directly from one sexual partner to another. Children, however, are particularly susceptible to sickness resulting from their parents' inappropriate behavior. Swelling in any part of the body, although most specifically the abdomen, is generally associated with sexually transmitted disease (Beaglehole and Beaglehole 1938, 285–86). A married couple with children avoid having intercourse in their sleeping house not for reasons of modesty but rather because their children might have contact with secretions remaining in the mats and thus contract "illness and limb swelling" (Beaglehole and Beaglehole 1938, 286).

Hereditary ulcers and swellings in certain Pukapukan families are attributed to the improper use of lovers' gifts. A man's children, for example, will become ill if he allows them to eat gifts of food from his mistress (Beaglehole and Beaglehole 1938, 292).

The second restriction on sexual conduct is that it should not take place between kinsmen within a three- to four-generation range of relationships. If kinsmen who are too closely related have sexual intercourse or marry, swelling sickness is often visited on succeeding generations by disgruntled ancestors. The families of one offending couple "prayed to their family gods to punish with sickness the terrible sin. The common punishment asked for was filiarial infection" of the miscreants and their descendants (Beaglehole and Beaglehole 1938, 262). It was suggested both to the Beagleholes in the 1930s and to me in the 1970s that families afflicted with filaria had a past history of misalliance.

Beyond sexual behavior, respect for others' property also figured importantly in the incidence of disease. Theft from land controlled by the three villages was particularly onerous. It was often punished by illness in various forms, including deafness, earache, constipation, urinary blockage, and perpetual hunger (Beaglehole and Beaglehole 1938, 310, 311, 313, 334). All prohibitions *(laui)* on land and its produce, whether village or family controlled, were strengthened by supernatural sanctions (Beaglehole and Beaglehole 1938, 32).

In addition to improper conduct, some conditions, such as that of diet, blood, and weather, affect susceptibility to disease.

While no one word directly translates as "health" or "healthy," *maloiloi* or *maloyi* 'strong' has important connotations of good health. In order to be strong, one must eat enough food and have enough blood. The Beagleholes reported that Pukapukans in the 1930s considered a man in good health to require a minimum of ten large drinking coconuts a day to remain strong (Beaglehole and Beaglehole 1938, 99). Prior et al. (1966) indicate that coconuts provided 36 percent of the total calories and over 75 percent of the fat calories in the Pukapukan diet. These figures may vary according to the availability of imported foods. Certain foods complement each other and satisfy hunger more quickly. Taro is particularly important in this regard; a charming folktale relates the story of a canoe of voracious voyagers who could not be satisfied until they reached an island sufficiently planted in taro (Beaglehole and Beaglehole n.d.).

The basic precept of Pukapukan diet is *na yangia koe?* 'Are you full? Have you had enough to eat?' Fatness is regarded as a hallmark of health and beauty. It is not clear if this is true to the point of extreme obesity; the physical requirements of the Pukapukan economy have probably always been such that there were few obese individuals (Prior et al. 1966).

There are certain dietary proscriptions relating to the sick. Sick persons may not eat fish, and in fact generally eat coconut. The "use of medicines is always accompanied by a tapu against the eating of fish until the sickness is completely cured. The tapu applies whether the disease treated is consumption or filaria. No rationalization could be given to account for the incompatibility of fish diet with medicines, but the rule is always rigidly enforced. To yield to a temptation to eat fish during convalescence is to cause a relapse" (Beaglehole and Beaglehole 1938, 342). While I am not sure if the tapu is as rigidly enforced today, sick persons appeared to restrict their diets considerably. The ban on fish may have something to do with a distinction between land and sea foods. It is remarkable, however, that parts of fish may be used in the manufacture of medicines; water in which the liver of a large, edible fish has been steeped may be used in the treatment of patients "grown thin and weak through prolonged illness" or of renal colic, according to the Beagleholes' primary informant (Beaglehole and Beaglehole 1938, 343).

A frequent explanation of ill health is that the sick person does not have enough blood *(e ye lava te toto)*. Blood is considered part of one's maternal inheritance and is closely associated with strength and life itself. Eating enough food, particularly taro, is thought to ensure sufficient blood.

Pukapukans today appear to believe that changing weather conditions can lead to illness. The phrase *tienanga o te reva,* a combination of the English *tienianga* 'change' and the Rarotongan *reva* 'climate' (Savage 1962), suggests that this idea may have been introduced since contact. Be it modern or of greater vintage, it accords with the traditional conservatism of Pukapukans in regard to the dangers of the outside world and increases their concern for their health when they venture into the different climates of Rarotonga and New Zealand. The theory that disease can be caused by variation in the weather may contribute to the Pukapukan practice of keeping stuffy, closed homes in Auckland.

DIAGNOSIS AND THERAPY

I have little information on diagnosis from my fieldwork in the 1970s. The Beagleholes' section on physical therapy is a good account of one practitioner's pharmacopoeia (Beaglehole and Beaglehole 1938, 342–43). Concoctions similar to those used in the 1930s appear to be used today. I would like, however, to raise a possible point of difference between the Beagleholes' and my own data on the subject of deep pressure massage in diagnosis and therapy.

The Beagleholes state that deep pressure massage is applied "over the seat of pain" or to the affected part (1938, 339), making no distinction between diagnosis and therapy. I observed one healer applying deep pressure to the ankles of a female client complaining of abdominal and back pain. The healer said he could diagnose by applying deep pressure to the ankles. This healer also diagnosed problems of the uterus (what the nurse said was a prolapsed uterus), which he treated by applying deep pressure to the abdomen and by prescribing a supportive bandage (which the patient only wore for a day, complaining it was as uncomfortable as the ailment).

If this case suggests a distinction between direct and indirect diagnosis, it may be particularly important in the treatment of women's ailments by male practitioners. The young woman who died of cancer while I was in Pukapuka had avoided the Cook Islands medical practitioner for as long as she could because of the nature of her complaint. Her abdomen was swelling; she knew she was not pregnant. Adolescents joked about her obviously "sexual" disease. She was embarrassed and did not want to be examined by the male doctor. In fact, the doctor suggested that he might have been able to do more for her had she let him examine her earlier. But the very direct nature of the western medical examination was an obstacle. Although both male and female healers in Pukapuka treat male and female clients, they do so in different ways depending on the nature of the complaint.

While I was in Pukapuka, I became aware of four males and one female who were recognized as healers. The Beagleholes mention that both men and women may be healers and that their practice does not differ substantially. Yet they also emphasize the importance of contact with the gods—a priestly, male function—in traditional diagnosis and therapy. It is noteworthy both that their stories of famous traditional healers are all about males and that only one of the five healers I encountered was female.

From discussions with the Cook Islands medical practitioner, I believe that these five healers may have been the principal practitioners for the entire population of 760, others practicing mostly within the confines of their own families. None of the five is solely occupied as a healer. One is a schoolteacher; the rest devote the majority of their time to subsistence cultivation and fishing and export some copra. The five healers are described in more detail in note 3. Healers are generally rewarded with small food gifts for their services; the prestige of the position is thought to be sufficient recompense and there are no set fees (Beaglehole and Beaglehole 1938, 335).

Traditionally, one became a healer through dream experience (Beaglehole and Beaglehole 1938, 334–35) and there was no hereditary transmission of knowledge. There may be, however, some sharing of recipes for the preparation of medicines. At least one kin group was recognized for its skill in healing: the major chiefly lineage on the island is referred to as "the lineage famed for healing the sick" in a love chant dating from the mid-nineteenth century ("Chant for a Sacred Maid," Beaglehole and Beaglehole n.d.).

While I made no systematic study of healing practices, massage and the prescription of coconut oil in various internal and externally applied preparations seemed to be the most frequent therapy. One healer treated me for gastrointestinal distress and for skin infections. The first distress he treated with deep pressure massage on the abdomen and a prescription of coconut oil. During the massage, he suggested that I would need to belch or expel gas; no mention was made of objects or spirits. The coconut oil served as a violent purgative. I drank about a quarter cup of it, followed by tinned peach juice as recommended by my household. I was up most of the night with nausea and diarrhoea. In the morning I was told to take a cold bath to stop the action of the oil and this worked fairly effectively. The effects of the coconut oil are said to be most extreme at first and then become moderated by regular use. I also took coconut oil internally for the skin sores.

The Cook Islands medical practitioner did not object to the practice of the Pukapukan healers within certain limits. He wished particularly that patients would come to see him first or at least concurrently. Given the general practice of deep pressure massage, his major concern was that the healers be aware that such massage was inappropriate in cases of appendicitis. Other cases, for which he could do little, he was in fact glad to refer to the healers for whatever relief they could provide.

CONCLUSION

Healthy living in traditional Pukapuka involved living within appropriate physical and social boundaries, and components of this belief system continue to affect contemporary attitudes and behavior. The threat to physical boundaries came from outsiders approaching the island. These intrusions challenged the conservative rhythm of atoll society as well as threatened it with epidemic sicknesses.

The challenge to physical boundaries is fairly comprehensible, but the moral component of Pukapukan theories of disease may involve a direct collision with western medical models. Consequently this behavioral component is not always forthrightly expressed. Pukapukans know full well that disease caused by improper acts such as theft or disobeying an ancestor and brought on by the intervention of spiritual beings is not part of the western medical model.

But while Pukapukans have some understanding of the western medical model, they know much less about western folk models for the causation of disease, models which have considerably more in common with their own. Understanding that New Zealanders, Australians, and North Americans of European derivation also seek psychological relief, social support, and the re-integration of a social fabric rent by the disruption of disease or death, might encourage less bounded dialogue. We all might agree, as Joseph Conrad writes in *Lord Jim,* that "strictly speaking, the question is not how to get cured, but how to live."

NOTES

1. Research in the Cook Islands from August 1972 to June 1974 was supported by National Science Foundation Dissertation Research Grant No. GS35431. Further research with Pukapukans in Auckland was undertaken while I taught at the University of Auckland during 1976. The University of Hawaii Department of Anthropology National Institutes of Mental Health Grant No. 5T32 MH15741 provided partial support during the writing of this chapter.

I would like to express my gratitude for the help of Pukapukans in the Cook Islands and in New Zealand. Very little of the story of how they approach health and illness is told here; perhaps someone will be inspired to record it in more detail.

When I studied in the Cook Islands in 1972–74, one of my major concerns was avoiding disease, not studying it. Yet, as I worked back over field notes and journals devoted primarily to the topics of kinship and social organization, I found occasional notes on cases of illness and therapy. These glimpses, together with published research by Ernest and Pearl Beaglehole and Ian Prior, have aided in the writing of this chapter. It is, I regret, notably short on indigenous terms for health and disease concepts and on detailed description of diagnosis and therapy.

The field research in Pukapuka involved a typical round of language learning, focused and less-structured interviews, and participant observation both at the village and island community level and within the household and neighborhood where I lived. At one point or another I interviewed members of virtually all households on the island. In addition, I conducted in-depth discussion and question-and-answer sessions with a group of eight Pukapukans, all age sixty-two or older.

2. I noticed that many inland house sites in Pukapuka appeared to have been deserted and asked what had motivated people to abandon these inland neighborhoods. Informants said that many people had severe skin diseases during the latter half of the nineteenth century and had moved from further inland to habitations on the lagoon front where they had easier access to the soothing water.

3. The first healer was a fifty-seven-year-old male who performed the deep pressure diagnosis on the ankles described above. He was a Cook Islands Christian Church member, had spent his entire life on the atoll, except for a year on Nassau, and had never married. He was a member of Roto village.

The second healer was a seventy-four-year-old male who had originally been known as a midwife. These skills are less often called into use now that there is a nurse-midwife stationed on the atoll. He had spent a year and a half on Nassau, a year in Aitutaki in the Lower Cooks, two years in Rarotonga, and almost two years in New Zealand. He was formerly a Cook Islands Christian Church member but converted to Roman Catholicism as an adult. He was married twice during the 1920s, and was twice divorced. He was a Ngake villager and lived only a few houses away from my household, whose members often consulted him.

The third healer was a sixty-four-year-old male who had spent eight and a half years in Rarotonga. He was a remarried widower and a Cook Islands Christian Church member. Perhaps because he lived in the furthest village, Yato, I was not aware of his practice until the Cook Islands medical practitioner mentioned him to me.

The fourth healer was a thirty-year-old male from the Lower Cook Group. He had lived in Pukapuka for eight years, married a Pukapukan woman, and was raising a young family. He attended the young woman who died and was the one who determined that her grandmother was the cause of her illness. He was Roman Catholic and a member of Ngake village. Although he was closely associated with our household, I was not aware of his practice until he treated me about a year after my arrival.

The fifth healer was a twenty-five-year-old unmarried female. She had spent a year and a half in Rarotonga and two years in Nassau. She belonged to the Cook Islands Christian Church and the village of Roto. She was very active as a healer in the neighborhood where I lived. I was most aware of her practice with women, especially younger ones, but she treated men as well. Some of her pharmacopoeia may have been of foreign origin. For example, I noted that she treated one young woman's menstrual distress with a concoction of coconut oil and crushed breadfruit leaves applied to the back. Breadfruit was only recently introduced to Pukapuka and is not plentiful.

It may be noteworthy that no Seventh Day Adventists are numbered among the healers of whom I was aware. Their religious beliefs may lead them to deal with illness in some other ways. Seventh Day Adventists form about 10 percent of the population, Roman Catholics another 14 percent, and Cook Islands Christian Church members the remaining 76 percent.

9

Tahitian Healing

Antony Hooper

Several of the earliest European voyagers in Tahiti, in spite of their difficulties with the local language and the many distractions which attended their visits, made observations of the common sicknesses and some of the local methods used for their treatment. Banks, who was on Tahiti and several islands of the neighboring Leeward group for nearly four months in 1769, mentions priestly "ceremonies for the cure of sick people" and was impressed by the apparent skill of local surgeons and the Tahitians' use of both "vulnerary herbs" and medicinal plants (Beaglehole 1962, 1:374–76). James Morrison, who enjoyed a longer and much more intimate contact with the people a decade or so later, wrote a fairly extensive account of the practices of mediums and the ideas on which their activities were based. He also mentions the Tahitians' surgical skills, although he had a poor opinion of the medicines which were used. He wrote that "for any mixed Complaint they have no remedy except it is applyd by Chance tho they always administer Some Medicine with their prayers . . ." (1935, 228).

European contact intensified during the closing decades of the eighteenth century and led to the extensive transformation of Tahitian society during the next twenty years. But whatever else the Tahitians took from Europeans (and they took over much in the way of both ideas and material goods) it is evident that they did not abandon the use of their own medical techniques—in spite of Ellis's somewhat rosy statement that such heathen practices had "entirely ceased" (1853, 3:44). Brodie was to note a few years later the people's "strange superstition that almost any of their wild herbs is preferable to European physic" (n.d., 10:11), and there are numerous references in missionary journals and letters to the activities of native mediums and curers. Pearse's account of events in his Leeward Islands parish during 1878 is particularly vivid and full.

We expelled nine members one month for involving themselves in superstitious practices. One of them was a deacon of the church and the others were relatives. There had been much sickness in the family and several had died. Through the leaven of heathen superstition still lurking in them, they were possessed of the idea that evil spirits still residing in the bones of their ancestors, were the cause of their afflictions. They resolved to burn the bones in order to destroy the power of the spirits. They also consulted the native sorcerer who confirmed them in their determination. But there was the difficulty of knowing the place where the bones were interred. They suspected that they were interred in the vicinity of their old marae, but the sorcerer told them he could discover the place. On the day appointed the relatives were conducted by him to the heathen marae of their ancestors, and after certain preliminaries he told them the place to dig. They at once set to work at the place indicated, and about a foot below the ground discovered a stone receptacle containing human bones, stones cut to the shape of human skulls, stone images, one like a dog, another a fowl, another a rat, another a lizard, another a fish etc. These were all taken out by the sorcerer who after performing certain incantations cast them into a large fire. . . . While speaking of superstition I will give you another form of it which is very common among certain families. It came to my knowledge as a case of church discipline at Tahaa. A member of a family was taken very ill native medicine failed to cure. In their distress they sent for the native sorcerer or diviner. On his arrival, after repeating certain formulae, he asked the relatives to confess to him for whose sin the sufferer was possessed by an evil spirit. One after another denied having sinned against him. At last one confessed having thought ill of him in his heart. This was considered to be the cause of the illness. Upon this confession the sorcerer based his conjurations and prayers, in order that the evil spirit may be exorcised. Certain ceremonies were also performed in pressing upon the body to know the position of the demon within, this being found, a gradual pressure of the hands on that part force the demon downward to the leg and forward to the foot so that he may escape. Thus being expelled from the sufferer, he is supposed to be cured and is expected to recover. As a rule medicine is also given, but if the recovery is effected, the cure is credited to the sorcery and not to the medicine. There is no doubt that the very faith in the enchantments often helps to restore. If the patient does not recover, the sorcerer is not blamed, for he avows that the cause whereby the sufferer became possessed was not revealed to him, for had it been, he would certainly have recovered. Thus often ill feeling is produced in the family, one accusing the other of being the cause of his affliction and death. When I was at Huahine some few months since we expelled several members for applying to the sorcerers, rather than trusting to God. It is strange that so much faith is placed in these superstitions.

Pearse appeared to be resigned to the view that only "true knowledge of the gospel" would overturn the power of these superstitions and "lead the people to trust in God and to the proper treatment of medicine . . ." (1878).

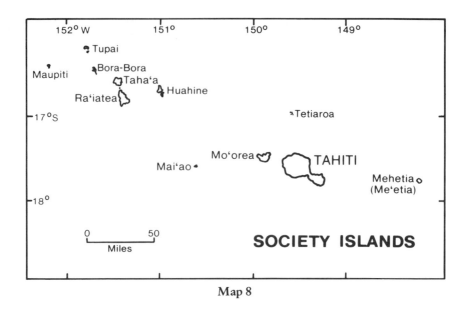

Map 8

This has not been the case. Both the Gospel and the Tahitians' belief in their local methods of curing have flourished during the century since Pearse wrote. Far from one having driven out the other, both are now an integral part of the distinctively Tahitian way of life. This has been pointed out by several writers, and in the scattered, uneven descriptive literature on the twentieth century Society Islands there are a number of brief accounts of indigenous medical practices. For the most part, these either describe various herbal remedies (Goupil 1926; Petard 1948; Salmon 1955) or recount exploits of well-known local healers (R. V. 1925; Sasportas 1924; Walker 1925). A recent article by Panoff (1966) is made up mostly of recipes for herbal remedies, making only a brief mention of what he terms *maladies surnaturelles*. Levy, on the other hand, has written perceptively (1967; 1973) about Tahitian concepts of the supernatural and the techniques used for the treatment of "supernatural maladies," making only passing reference to the use of herbal remedies.

In this chapter I take a somewhat different perspective on these topics. Although I describe several herbal remedies in some detail I am not here concerned with their possible pharmacological properties or physiological effects; and although I give several accounts of the treatment of "ghost sicknesses" I cannot, as Levy does, point up the psychodynamic principles which might be involved. My perspective here is more directly ethnographic, beginning with the Tahitian concept of *ma'i* 'sickness', and attempting to describe the associated ideas and practices. I begin with an account of the Tahitian cultural system for labeling and classifying disorders, together with some of the explanatory principles which are involved. I then describe the therapeutic practices in common use. The concluding section suggests some relationships between these ideas and practices and certain features of rural Tahitian social structure.

This account is based upon data gathered during the 1960s by field research in two rural communities in the Iles sous-le-vent,[1] a group of five high islands and four atolls to the northwest of Tahiti, the largest island and metropolitan center of French Polynesia. In these islands, outside of one small urban center on the island of Ra'iatea, the population is dominantly Polynesian, living in small communities on the coastal fringes of the larger volcanic islands. They speak of themselves as *mā'ohi* 'indigenous' or *ta'ata Tahiti* 'Tahitians', and see themselves and their way of life as distinct from that of the other ethnic groups, metropolitan French, *demi* and Chinese, who make up the population of the Territory. This distinctiveness is made of many elements—race, language, and religious affiliation as well as a whole body of customs and practices relating to land, kinship, preferred foods, and the life cycle. Among these practices we may also place the system of folk medicine described here, which exists alongside the fairly good facilities—small hospitals, and dressing stations staffed by government-trained medical personnel—which are located within reach of the rural people and are freely available to them. Rural Tahitians have a mixed attitude toward these services, regarding them with abhorrence, envy, and fear of their injections and surgical procedures. Generally only the most serious cases are taken for this sort of treatment.

There is no vestige remaining of the elaborate nineteenth-century Tahitian polity or the ideas of inherited rank on which it was based. There are neither titles nor "chiefs" apart from those who are elected to serve as minor administrative officials in the districts into which the rural areas are divided. Executive government is under the direction of an appointed French governor, although the local Territorial Assembly (elected by universal suffrage) has for the past twenty years given strong expression to local as against metropolitan French interests. All Tahitians are highly involved in the market economy of the Territory; on Tahiti itself many are engaged in wage labor, and even in the most remote rural areas the money gained from the sale of cash crops forms an essential part of domestic household economies.

MAJOR CATEGORIES OF SICKNESS

The Tahitian term which I gloss as "sickness" is *ma'i*. All forms of plant and animal life may be *ma'i* 'sick', or *pohe ma'i* 'overcome with sickness', although it is only the *maʻi* suffered by human beings which is the subject of any conceptual elaboration. Tahitians speak of injuries to animals with the same terms that are used to refer to human injuries, and while they do not discount the possibility that domestic and other animals may suffer from "ghost sickness" I did not learn of any specific examples. Sick animals are seldom cared for in any way, and there are no specialists for their treatment; those suffering from anything more obscure than the most obvious injury are passed off as merely having "dog sickness" or "chicken sickness" and are left to recuperate, or to die.

Tahitians commonly distinguish four major kinds of *maʻi*, three of which are labeled by separate *parau rahi,* or "general terms." At this level of generality the contrasts are based on the different presumed causes of the sicknesses. In many instances, however, an explicit distinction is made between an immediate or effective cause and the underlying or final cause. In general discourse, these levels and contrasts are clear from the particular contexts. Tahitians in general, even those who specialize to some extent as curers, are not given to elaborating taxonomic or typological niceties at this level.

The first major category of *maʻi* includes all those events which would be classified in English as "injuries"—sprains, breaks, cuts, burns, and so forth. Each specific type of injury may be labeled by a specific term, as is the case in English, although there is no single Tahitian term for the category as a whole. When speaking of particular cases, people will ordinarily use the appropriate term for the specific type of injury, and the question of a category corresponding to the English "injury" does not arise. In discussing the taxonomic status of particular injuries (such as *mutu* 'cut' or *paʻapaʻa* 'burn'), however, informants would not accept them as belonging in any of the other three major categories, preferring to speak of them all together as a separate category which they defined by straightforward listing of the component items—"bruises, cuts and that sort of thing . . ."

I shall use, then, the English term "injury" for this unlabeled category. For Tahitians, as for ourselves, the immediate cause of any injury is usually seen as either obvious or readily inferred without requiring any diagnostic skill. It is this feature which sets off the category from other categories such as "true sickness" and "ghost sickness." At the level of ultimate causes, however, a particular injury may be readily accepted as being also an instance of "ghost sickness."

The crucial issue here is the notion of "accident." Tahitians have the notion that many things happen simply by chance, and that some injuries may be caused simply by misadventure, and lack of adequate care or supervision. But they are, at the same time, also very ready to try and discern, behind the apparently fortuitous circumstances of an injury, some underlying meaning or cause. It is the classic question of what brought about the particular set of circumstances surrounding the "accident." The answer may, in appropriate circumstances, be provided by beliefs about the actions and propensities of "ghosts." The tendency to seek for such underlying meanings and causes seems to be most marked when either the injury or the surrounding circumstances are at all unusual. There was, for example, a lame youth in the community whose disability was due to a complex fracture of a femur which he had suffered as a child when he fell through a hole in a wooden house-floor. I was told that people were at the time surprised by the seriousness of the break when the child had suffered such a comparatively short fall; and when the local treatments did not work as expected, the injury was interpreted as the work of a "ghost" which had pulled his leg through the hole with particular viciousness and force.

Again, it is very commonly believed that certain activities, such as fishing, are particularly dangerous if they are undertaken on a Sunday or other holy day; such activities are liable to be punished with attack by sharks or other misadventures, and appropriate cases seem to be always readily available to support this contention. The punishment in these cases seems to be conceived of as taking place automatically, without the intervention of any active being or agency, but when pressed for further explanation most people will say that they suppose that it must be God's doing.

This kind of explanation derives its particular force from some very basic, widely held, and apparently deep-seated Tahitian ideas about the nature of sickness and health in general, which I shall discuss in the concluding section.

Ma'i mau 'true sickness' is a second major category, which may be distinguished from "injury" both by intrinsic nature and the lack of any obviously identifiable effective cause. True sickness may *tupu noa* 'just grow' upon a person who has formerly enjoyed good health, and is seen as being due to something which comes from outside the body rather than arising from within the body itself. The intrinsic nature and immediate effective cause of *ma'i mau* is not a topic on which Tahitians are prone to speculate in any serious way. They see it as a worldwide phenomenon which has been present at least since biblical times, and having no special manifestations among Tahitians as distinct from other peoples. For this reason, they will readily offer what French names for disease they may know as being exact translations of Tahitian terms, and they see their own herbal remedies as working in precisely the same way as the potions, pills, and injections which are available from the French pharmacies and hospital services. It is believed, however, that people who are *puta to'eto'e* (lit. "pierced by cold" or "chilled") or *puta mahana* 'pierced by the sun' have a weakened bodily resistance and are prone to succumb to any variety of true sickness. Diet is also seen to play a part in resistance to this category of sickness. The general feeling of satiety and well-being denoted by the term *pa'ia* is said by adults to be only truly attained from meals of fish, coconut sauce, and local vegetable foods. Canned foods, in spite of the extent to which they are in fact used in the rural areas, are held to be unsatisfying; there is even speculation that they are the cause of cancer. And many Tahitians will argue that their ancestors in the days before they ate "foreign" foods extensively, were much healthier than the people are at the present time. As evidence for this fact they point to the skulls which are secreted in well-known rock crevices, which all have well-preserved teeth.

"Ghosts" and ghostly influences are not seen as causing true sickness in any way. A "ghost sickness" may, however, be mistaken for one of the varieties of true sickness and its real nature thus not discovered until it is seen that herbal treatments are having no effect, and a specialist in the treatment of ghost sickness has been consulted. A diagnosis of ghost sickness by a specialist then leads to a complete reclassification of the sickness and a radical change in the method of treatment.

Ghosts may, however, be involved in other ways with those who are inflicted with one of the varieties of true sickness. A young man who was said to have been chilled by an extensive period spent spearfishing in deep waters off the barrier reef, fell quite severely sick; it was thought that he had a true sickness and several kinds of herbal remedies were tried over a period of several days. As the youth's condition worsened, a specialist was called upon. He confirmed the original diagnosis of a true sickness as being correct, but stated that there were special subsequent complications due to the fact that the ghost of the patient's dead mother had great *aroha* 'compassion' and wanted him to rest with her in death so that he could be relieved of his suffering. For these circumstances there seemed to be little that could be done. Herbal treatments were continued, and the boy's father visited the grave of his dead wife to plead with her ghost to allow a recovery to take place. Only when the patient was very severely ill was he taken to hospital, where he died a day later—probably of pneumonia.

True sickness is the only major category of *ma'i* which embraces an extensive number of named varieties, each of which may in turn be composed of a number of named subvarieties. The principles of classification at this level are both elusive and obscure, and I shall deal with them in greater detail in the following section.

The Tahitian term which I translate as "ghost" is *tūpāpa'u,* and an understanding of the nature of *ma'i tūpāpa'u* 'ghost sickness' involves a description of some distinctively Tahitian concepts. The great majority of

Tahitians are Christian, and have been for generations. The Christian concepts of "soul" and "spirit" are translated in the Tahitian Bible as *vārua,* and, invariably, the nature of *vārua* is seen in more or less strictly biblical terms. The *vārua* is seen as being given to each child, by God, either at birth or at some point during its gestation, and is taken by God again at death—usually to Heaven. (Most Tahitians say that they believe in Hell in fairly literal terms, but they seem to doubt whether there are in fact many Tahitians there.)

It is widely believed that each person has "within" him a *tūpāpa'u*—an incorporeal *mea* 'thing' which can leave the body during dreams and which survives the body's death, going neither to Heaven nor to Hell. As informants explain it, the *tūpāpa'u* is "without a body, like the air or a shadow." The relationship between these two concepts, the Christian notion of *vārua* and the local one of *tūpāpa'u*, is an interesting one. In discussing the nature of "life" and "death" Tahitians use a fairly literal biblical idiom, seeing *ora* 'life' and the *vārua* as coming ultimately from God, whereas the *tūpāpa'u* on the other hand are seen as "just there." When talking about these matters once with me, an elderly Protestant deacon who took pleasure in toying with such ideas carefully explained the nature of both concepts. Then, in reply to my question as to whether he had both a *vārua* and a *tūpāpa'u* "inside" him, he replied with a laugh, "Perhaps I do, but perhaps there is only one thing, and sometimes it is a *vārua* and sometimes it is a *tūpāpa'u*. How can we know such things?" For him, as for most other Tahitians, there is no real conflict between the two sets of belief. The concepts simply belong to different universes of discourse. While I never heard any Tahitian be sceptical about *vārua,* a few people (in my experience usually men) would voice some skepticism about the reality of *tūpāpa'u,* saying that they were the creation of one's thoughts only, and that if you didn't believe in them you would never see them. Such statements did not, however, seem to blunt in any way their fascination for stories about *tūpāpa'u.*

In spite of this occasional vein of skepticism, most of the Tahitian explanations which I heard about the nature of *tūpāpa'u,* as well as stories about their exploits, showed that there is a widely shared and consistent body of beliefs about them. *Tūpāpa'u* have the physical and personality characteristics of the living person, being either male or female, aggressive or retiring, and so forth. Although they leave a living body at, or shortly after, the body's death, they will tend to remain in the vicinity of where the body is buried. They are capable of instant movement and have been known to make journeys to distant lands. *Tūpāpa'u* watch over the affairs of the living, especially those of their living kinsmen. For most Tahitians, the ghost of a kinsman is looked upon as being generally protective and not nearly so anxiety-provoking as an unrelated or unknown ghost. *Tūpāpa'u* are, however, vengeful, and occasionally capricious and playful in their relations with the living. Unlike *vārua*, which are never visible, *tūpāpa'u* may be seen by living people, to whom they appear to walk a few inches above the surface of the ground, often making a characteristic whistling sound. Dogs and other animals can often see or be aware of them even when humans remain oblivious to their presence. They are generally held to dislike sweet scents and perfumes, and, according to some informants, are afraid of bamboo.

Although Tahitians feel especially aware and afraid of *tūpāpa'u* when they are alone or in isolated, unfrequented places, it is not often that ghosts will appear, quite unprovoked, in such circumstances. The most common and important manifestation of *tūpāpa'u* is when they cause sickness. A *tūpāpa'u* may be the ultimate cause of an injury, and may be implicated in some instances of true sickness, as explained above. But there are also numerous occasions of sickness which are seen as due to direct *tūpāpa'u* influence and intervention. These sicknesses usually have a bizarre or frightening quality to them, and they can be cured only by specialist curers.

A fourth major category of sickness is known as *ma'i fa'autu'a*, literally "retribution sickness." From one point of view this may be seen as being a special variety of ghost sickness since it is also due to "supernatural" causes. In contrast to ghost sickness though, the supernatural agency at work is not a definite *tūpāpa'u* but is seen as a more abstract entity still, almost as a principle of Justice. Some informants state simply that it is the work of God. The essential feature of a *ma'i fa'autu'a* is that it is a punishment for wrongdoing—not an automatic punishment, since many wrongs are seen as never being punished, but one that is inherently just and proper.

It is in terms of these four major categories that rural Tahitians commonly speak about *ma'i* in general, and organize their perceptions and theories about particular instances of sickness. Both specialists and laymen may, however, disagree in their diagnoses, or change them according to circumstances. Diagnosis, and the social relationships involved in sickness and the curing process, form the subject of the following section.

DIAGNOSIS AND CURING

Ma'i is a subject of obvious and direct concern to all rural Tahitians, the most obvious reason for this being that their very livelihoods depend upon physical activity in gardening, tree climbing, and fishing. Ill health is not only personally inconvenient or distressing. It can tax, in a very rapid and direct manner, the livelihood and well-being of whole families. The state of health of community members is a constant and persistent

Tahitian Healing 167

item of everyday conversation, and even the most minor indisposition is closely watched and its progress inquired after, until it should become serious or else clear up completely. There is considerably more to this interest than idle curiosity or decent neighborly concern.

Injuries of one sort or another, although they may be alarming when they happen, are coped with in a fairly matter-of-fact and straightforward way. Cuts are generally tightly bound with pieces of ripped-up clothing to stop the flow of blood, occasionally with the addition of a few crushed leaves believed to have the property of making blood congeal. Scalds and superficial burns may be rubbed with butter, or, if none is immediately available, smeared with a soft mud which is allowed to dry in place. For scalds, many people recommend pressing a rotten leaf of 'ape (a taro-like plant which grows wild, Colocasia macrorrhisa Schott) onto the affected area. This is said to bring about a cure overnight, although it does have the unfortunate effect of irritating the surrounding unscalded skin. A widely known treatment for a child taken unconscious and drowning from the water is to place him head down over an adult's back with his legs over the adult's shoulders; the adult then runs with the child until the water "breaks" and consciousness returns. Broken bones are set (often rather approximately) in place and the limb or surrounding area coated with sticky breadfruit sap and bound with either cloth or *more*, a clothlike substance made from the bast of breadfruit bark. Practically all adults seem to know of straightforward first aid remedies of this kind, although many may be unwilling to take the responsibility of carrying them out. Whenever possible, the injured person is taken as quickly as possible to his or her home, where members of the family can take the decisions as to what should be done. Others may by sympathetic, but Tahitians are not effusive about shows of concern in such matters.

With *ma'i mau* 'true sickness', the onset is usually defined by the individual concerned. The adoption of a "sick role" in Tahiti involves a voluntary withdrawal from all or most ongoing activities—work, visiting, meetings, household duties, church, sport—and the patient's retiring to his usual house and resting. An individual is not expected to continue with normal activities at the cost of personal discomfort if he has declared himself as *ma'i*, and accusations of malingering are not common. At the early stages of sickness the responsibility for care and treatment is wholly on family and household members. It is not customary for anyone other than these people to visit the sick person, inquire directly about symptoms, or to offer advice of any kind. Members of the immediate family, especially parents, may prepare an herbal remedy that they happen to know, or if the indisposition seems likely to be more than a passing one, to seek out the advice of a semispecialist in such treatments.

Most adult women who have cared for small children know several recipes for "small medicines" or "children's medicines" which they will make up and give to their children when they are indisposed, without feeling that they should consult anyone else on the matter. Many have considerable trust in their "own" remedies as being clearly the most suitable for their own children, and one woman told me that she had used only one remedy to cure all of the ills which her son had suffered from in childhood.

The treatment of sickness in adults is seen as a somewhat more complex and serious matter, and the advice of a *tahu'a* is more readily sought. *Tahu'a* is a term with a fairly wide range of referents. In its widest sense it refers to a person with specialist skills of any sort, particularly when that person is performing a directive role in some undertaking. The term is still occasionally used in this wider sense in the rural areas (I have heard it used to refer to both a boatbuilder and a Protestant pastor) but it is a somewhat archaic usage. More commonly, a *tahu'a* is a "curer" and the term may be used with or without qualifiers to designate a special field of competence. A *tahu'a rā'au* is one who specializes in the use of *rā'au* 'medicines' for curing, *rā'au* being the generic Tahitian term for "plants" and also for "medicines" of both European or local origin. *Tahu'a rā'au* is, however, never used to refer to a European-trained doctor, who is always known as a *taote,* a nineteenth-century Tahitian rendering of the English "doctor."

A person who simply knows a few "medicines" and even uses them freely to aid both members of the family and neighbors, is not referred to as a *tahu'a* for that reason. The term is reserved for those who make something of a specialty of diagnosis and have recourse to a number of medicines as well as the ability to concoct new ones. In the small community of about two hundred people which I knew best there were three people, two women and a man, who were known as *tahu'a rā'au*. Of these three, the man was held to be much more skilled and effective than the other two, who had, in fact, learned some of their prescriptions from him. One of the women specialized somewhat in the treatment of children's complaints, and knew by heart perhaps a dozen prescriptions. The other, who was not very frequently consulted, had a special exercise book in which she had written down the prescriptions for sixty-nine named medicines. These entries were not ordered in any way, but represented notes which she had made over a period of years as she learned the medicines from various sources, both inside and outside the community. The man, who was widely held to be the only person in the community who *really* knew about *rā'au,* had never committed his knowledge to writing. During the period of nearly three weeks which he devoted to instructing me about *rā'au,* and during which we would work for three to four hours together every day, he did not refer at all to written notes. Other people in the community agreed with his own statement that the considerable body of prescriptions which he knew was held entirely in his memory. He was at the time a widower, living with his adopted children and their families, and was a mainstay of the community's Protestant church group, although he was not a deacon. The study of the Bible, together with a little of the less demanding garden work of the household and his work as a *tahu'a*, were his main occupations. His knowledge of medicines was gained mostly from his father, who had also been something of a *tahu'a* in his lifetime. But he also experimented with new prescriptions of his own, keeping those which proved to be effective.

During our daily sessions, he was confident and organized in his approach, patiently answering during the initial sessions all my questions concerning technical terms, and the names of plant parts which were new to me. We worked, at his direction, systematically through seven varieties of common *ma'i mau*, together with the thirty-two subvarieties which he distinguished. He gave me first a cursory description of the symptoms, followed by a list of ingredients for the appropriate *rā'au*, and then their method of preparation and the dosage to be followed.

The following is the verbatim account of his instructions for the *rā'au* for *tui hotete*, a variety of true sickness, and is a fair example of the way in which instructions for making *rā'au* are communicated orally between adults when it is presumed that the listener is familiar with the plants employed and the common techniques of preparation.

1. E piti rau'ere nono para, piti mea pu'u, 'aute e piti rau'ere.
2. Tāpū i te hō'ē ha'ari, vaiho te pape i roto i te 'āu'a, va'u te ha'ari i roto i te pape.
3. Pāpāhia 'āmui, pū'ohu.
4. Taviri i roto te ha'ari.
5. Tunu te 'ōfa'i 'ia 'ama, tu'u i roto i te 'āu'a.
6. Tāpo'i, e ia to'eto'e fa'ainu pauroa, hō'ē noa inura'a.

A fairly free translation of the six sections follows.

1. Two mature *nono* leaves, two immature ones, two *'aute* leaves.
2. Cut a [fully mature] coconut, put the liquid into a bowl, grate the meat of the coconut into this liquid.
3. Pound up [the leaves] together, wrap them in cloth.
4. Wring [the bundle of leaves so that the liquid runs out] into the coconut water.
5. Heat [a small] stone until hot, place it in the bowl.
6. Cover, and when it is cold give it to be drunk, all at once.

In the treatment of patients, a process which might last several weeks and involve daily visits, the medicines would always be made under the direction of the *tahu'a,* either by his adopted daughter or by a member of the patient's family, with any willing hands being pressed into the collection of the plant ingredients. The plants used in medicines are generally of no commercial value; many, in fact, are regarded otherwise as weeds and they are taken freely from anyone's land.

Rā'au, however, are regarded as personal property. Even though the prescription may be a simple one, learned and committed to memory within a matter of minutes, it remains the property of an owner, whether that person is a *tahu'a* or not, and should not be made except under his or her direction. Failure to do so is widely believed to result in the medicine being *ma'au* 'spoiled' and rendered ineffectual. There appears to be no clear doctrine as to the way in which the injury takes place, but most people believe it is due to the action of ghosts. For what are apparently very similar reasons, there should be direct and continuing contact between patient and *tahu'a* during the process of treatment, since medicines made in one place and taken to a patient some distance away are liable to be *'īāhia* 'stolen' by ghosts while in transit. As it was explained to me, "One opens the bundle with the crushed medicine in it, and there is nothing there at all!"

Recipes for medicines may, however, be *hōro'ahia* 'given' by one person to another. This appears to be done quite frequently by people who have no pretensions to being *tahu'a* when they simply get weary of the business of making up a medicine for a particular patient. *Tahu'a* do not commonly give prescriptions in this fashion, maintaining that they become *ma'au* simply by the transaction, and they are then put to the trouble of having to concoct new prescriptions as replacements.

It is clear that these beliefs all serve to define *tahu'a* as a distinct social role. The only other kind of special knowledge which is regarded in a somewhat similar light by rural Tahitians is that having to do with the traditional songs and dances, which are regarded as being the property of the individuals or groups who created them. But there is here no explicit connection with ghosts or ideas of spoilage. Most other kinds of special knowledge, particularly those having to do with fishing and gardening, are very jealously guarded against others who try, either openly or by trickery, to find it out.

Medicines are never bought and sold among Tahitians and the *tahu'a* who use them maintain an ideology of completely free services to all who should ask for them. There is no ethic that they should be given gifts in appreciation of their services, although gifts are in fact sometimes given, even in the form of money. In general, the attitude to true sickness and the various remedies available is strictly pragmatic. If the medicines known by one person fail to bring about a cure it is expected that others, whether *tahu'a* or not, will be asked to help.

There are no particular herbal ingredients of *rā'au* which are regarded as being specific in their effects, or as being especially indicated by certain symptoms. The commonly held view is that there are some plants which have "always" been known by Tahitians to have curative properties, as distinct from others which have no particular effects. Some thoughtful informants put forward the view that all plants may well have useful curing properties, but many of them are not known simply because they have not been tried. It is generally thought that the curing plants are there by God's good grace, for Tahitians to learn about and to use. Most of them are thought to be *rā'au mā'ohi* 'native plants', although they may be used to cure the ailments of anyone, not only Tahitians. *Popa'ā* 'Europeans' have their plants and their medicines as well, which are held to be no better or worse on the whole than *rā'au Tahiti* 'Tahitian medicines'.

However, in spite of the lack of any doctrine concerning the specific properties of curing plants, Tahitians do not regard it as proper to make up a recipe containing extracts from all the curing plants and administer it to a patient. When I raised this possibility I was firmly told that "it simply wasn't done that way." Yet, in certain unusual circumstances, this is precisely what is done. Before leaving the community on a six-month labor contract in the Tuamotu group, a young man took the precaution of asking the *tahu'a rā'au* to supply him with a bottle of *rā'au rahi,* literally a "large medicine," but as he described it to me "one with a lot of different things in it." He wanted it, he said, because he didn't know if there would be a good *tahu'a* where he would be working, or even if the necessary plants would be available; and he used the medicine something like a tonic, drinking a little at regular intervals or whenever he felt indisposed in any way.

In marked contrast to the complexity and precision of the recipes for Tahitian medicines, the recognized symptoms and the syndromes indicating particular, named true sicknesses appear relatively vague and imprecise. Consider, for example, my informant's description of the indications for the eight named subvarieties of the true sickness known as *ira:*

1. *Ira miti.* Found characteristically in children, who feel sick and have a fever at ten in the morning and feel better at two in the afternoon; *miti* in Tahitian means "sea water," and there is held to be a connection between these symptoms and the diurnal movements of the tide. (Lunar tidal movements are barely noticeable in the Society Islands.)
2. *Ira vaeha'a.* A pain on one side of the face only, which may occur in both children and adults.

3. *Ira 'āhure*. Inflammation and breaking of the skin around the urethra of female children.
4. *Ira tui*. A discharge of pus and matter from the ears, and a lot of matter in the eyes.
5. *Ira 'ute*. Red, painful lips in children.
6. *Ira nīnamu*. Occurs only in children, the symptoms being darkened lips and eyes, fever, headache, and desire for sleep.
7. *Ira hitirere*. Known also as *ira hui*. Startling in young children. The same medicine is used as for *ira ninamu*.
8. *Hua ira*. A swelling of a child's penis, associated with inflammation, and, sometimes, a darkening of the skin.

Two features of this description might seem puzzling—to both medical specialists and those who, like myself, are innocent of any specialized medical knowledge. The first is the recognition of some unusual and apparently bizarre symptoms, such as the waning and waxing of the fever which is held to indicate *ira miti*. My informant maintained that he did not know the precise way in which the tides influenced the course of this particular illness, although he had seen several cases of it, all of which he had been able to cure. The qualifying terms used to indicate the other subcategories of *ira* are all comparatively straightforward and descriptive. *Vaeha'a* 'side' refers to the characteristic location of the pain; *'āhure* 'turned inside out' refers to the exposure of the urethra; *tui* is somewhat more complex since it refers in this instance to another category of true sickness which is characterized by swellings due to accumulations of pus and matter; and this category is, in turn, related to *tui* meaning a boil located in the neck region; *'ute* is a shortened form of *'ute'ute* 'red' and in this case simply describes the condition of the lips; *nīnamu* 'dark blue' again describes the characteristic symptom, as does *hitirere* 'to start, move suddenly, as by surprise'; *hua* 'genitals' refers to the location of the malady.

The second and somewhat more puzzling question is what features these separate sicknesses are believed to share in common. What makes them all instances of the category *ira*? The term *ira* has two somewhat distinct meanings in Tahitian. Besides the category of true sickness, it refers to a mole or some sort of permanent discoloration, such as a birthmark, on the skin. Most informants see the two uses of the term as homonyms; others are not prepared to be so definite, pleading ignorance of the old (and, by implication, true) meanings. No informant, however, considered either moles or birthmarks to be any sort of sickness, true or otherwise; they are regarded as being things that are "just there." I was never able to obtain a satisfactory or coherent account, from *tahu'a rā'au* or others, of the "true nature" of *ira,* or even what they saw as the features common to all its manifestations. My informants came to share my puzzlement, but not my concern. They regarded the question as valid enough, but hardly saw it as an absorbing one. None of the other categories of true sickness presents quite the same difficulties. My *tahuʻa* informant was explicit about the fact that fever, red swellings, and discoloration are characteristic of all manifestations of the category of *māriri*, and also that all varieties of *tui* are due to accumulations of pus and matter in the head region. Similarly, *heʻa* appears to have connotations of dryness associated with all of its manifestations.

Ira is apparently more obscure than any of these other categories of true sickness, but I am reluctant to see it as being an entirely miscellaneous category—especially as it has been defined in a recent dictionary[2] as a "catégorie de maladie qui comprend entre autres des maux de tete et des convulsions." *Ira* appears to have the following distinctive features. It is found characteristically in children, and affects both the head and the external urinary organs. If we overlook for the moment the enigmatic symptoms of *ira miti,* and accept that *ira hitirere* 'startling' could be readily associated with a disorder of the eyes (since the startling movement might be interpreted as the child "seeing" something which is in fact not there), then the manifestations of *ira* in the head all involve either headaches or disorders of the eyes or lips. This feature of *ira* would then explain the subcategory *ira tui,* which is unusual in that the qualifying term *tui* also refers to a separate category of true sickness associated with swellings and discharges of pus, but not usually with matter in the eyes as is the case with *ira tui*. The special features of *ira miti* remain unexplained. Tahitians do not to my knowledge see any other special influences of the tide on either human beings or the natural world, although it is known to influence the movements of fish, particularly on reefs and in the lagoons.

In the light of this brief descripton of some diagnostic criteria, it is hardly surprising that Tahitians should hold the view that the diagnosis of sickness is a difficult and imprecise matter, in which even specialists are liable to make mistakes. Although *maʻi* is a very frequent topic of conversation (like crops, fishing, weather, and the movements of other people) in the daily round of gossip and casual encounter, the interest is always in individual cases and the particular people called upon to help. Questions of prognosis and etiology are the dominant concerns; diagnosis is left to the *tahuʻa*.

Tahuʻa rāʻau, and also any others who might be called upon to make up a medicine which they know, are guided in only a very general way by the visible symptoms and the patient's statements about feeling states. A few minutes of inquiry and conversation are all that is taken in most cases, before a particular medicine has been decided upon and helpers instructed to gather the necessary ingredients. Even at this point, people do not commonly either inquire about or discuss an appropriate name for the sickness. If, after a day or so of treatment with a particular medicine there has been no improvement, the medicine may be changed—and this process may be repeated over a period of several weeks with a half dozen or so different treatments, until one is found that is associated with some recovery. This medicine may then be used to define the sickness.

When I commented on the apparent arbitrariness of this procedure I was told by my *tahu'a* informant that it was really no different from that followed by European *taote* 'doctors', and he went on to describe several instances he knew of where Tahitian hospital patients had been treated with various medicines until the right one was found which could effect a cure. Although his knowledge of these cases could have been only partial and based on inferences from very incomplete information, his statement nevertheless probably contains a certain element of truth. What western medical practitioner has not in fact modified his initial diagnosis on the grounds of the effectiveness, or lack of effect, of the remedies prescribed? However, while the observations may be true enough of the practices actually followed in many instances by western physicians, they hardly describe the procedures of the scientific or "biologistic" tradition of western medicine which seek to define disease strictly in terms of indicators of biological discontinuity and change.

This being so, there is an obvious contrast in the most basic procedures of the two systems of medical practice. In general terms the western biologistic medical tradition may be said to seek precise definitions of the nature of various diseases, and their appropriate cures. In the Tahitian system it is the cures and remedies which are the starting point, and the knowledge of how to concoct them which is organized, written down in many instances, and passed on. The two systems thus start from opposite poles, though they may find a common middle ground. Western medicine attempts to define diseases precisely and seek cures. Tahitian medical specialists start with the cures but are necessarily vague about the nature of the diseases, which can, in fact, be defined only by the cures which are found to be effective.[3]

A somewhat similar process of elimination may lead to suspicions that a particular case might not be one of true sickness at all. If medicines fail to effect any improvements in a patient's condition within the expected time, or if an illness should take any dramatic, severe, or unexpected turn, this is commonly held to be an indication of *ma'i tūpāpa'u* 'ghost sickness'. The diagnosis of *ma'i tūpāpa'u* cannot, however, be confirmed without consultation with a specialist *tahu'a* who commands techniques for communicating with ghosts. Such *tahu'a* may be distinguished by various terms, of which *tahu'a hi'ohi'o*[4] is probably the most general.

At the time I did my field research there were no active *tahu'a hi'ohi'o* in either of two communities in which I lived. There was, however, one elderly man, whom I shall call Fatu, who had a reputation of having been a powerful *tahu'a* in the recent past, before he became *paruparu* 'weak' and, as others said of him, *fa'aruehia e tona tūpāpa'u* 'abandoned by his ghost [familiar]'. Fatu's description of how he acquired his powers is an interesting one. He was born on a neighboring island and adopted to his father's kin in a community a short distance away from his present house. While he was a young man, when he and his wife were working as sharecroppers on land owned by another, several of their children died in infancy. No *tahu'a* seemed to be able to save them. After the death of their fifth infant, Fatu went off by himself one evening to a corner of his house and privately asked his parents and his grandparents to come and help him cure his children. He described this act as not a *pure* 'prayer' but just an "asking in his thoughts." He then heard the noise of a cricket (an omen commonly associated with messages from absent kinsmen) before he fell into a light sleep and felt a hand laid on his arm. He woke and saw before his eyes a whole group of *tūpāpa'u*—his parents, grandparents, and many others, all of whom were *feti'i* 'cognatic kin'. He asked who among them was their leader and was told that it was the grandfather of his adoptive mother whom he remembered as having been a very old man when he was a young child. So he asked this *tūpāpa'u* to "come inside him" and help him save his children. At this stage Fatu did not want the power to cure people generally, and was concerned only for his own children, but when people round about learned of his new powers they started bringing sick people to him for diagnosis and cure. Since his wife was an accomplished *tahu'a rā'au* they had between them a flourishing practice for many years. Fatu was brought to his present home by the father of a girl patient whom he had cured of a ghost sickness, and then sought to adopt. When I knew him he was a widower who lived alone in a small house on the inland border of the community, cared for by neighbors, the adopted daughter and her parents, and by his own children who would visit from time to time from a neighboring community. He was an industrious gardener, quiet and humorous in manner, though given to displays of dancing and shouting on the very rare occasions when he could obtain enough liquor to get drunk. Most people in the community had been somewhat in awe of him, and slightly afraid, when he was in full possession of his powers, but they now could regard him with a friendly affection, and were rather proud to be able to tell of his exploits. As a somewhat frail old man, he was pleased to be left in peace and declared himself relieved that his *tūpāpa'u* did not visit him any more. He would still give medical advice, however, to close associates who sought his help.

In describing the acquisition and nature of his powers, Fatu emphasized that they came from the *tūpāpa'u* of his own ancestor working inside him, and were not *mea ho'o* 'bought things' like the powers of some other *tahu'a* who were, as he put it, *fa'aau matahiti* or "on a yearly arrangement." The distinction which he drew is a common one in Tahitian thought. Some *tahu'a* are held to derive their powers from an ancestral ghost who can be called upon to offer advice and to do supernatural deeds without any demands for repayment. Others, however, are said to have obtained their powers through a voluntary contract with a *tūpāpa'u* who is not a kinsman, and may be not even a Tahitian; these *tūpāpa'u* are of people who were, in real life, very powerful and influential. These *tahu'a* are believed to acquire their power to command the *tūpāpa'u* by rituals performed at disused pagan religious centers and involving a definite contract by which the *tahu'a* undertakes to pay for the power he has acquired by supernaturally killing one of his own close kinsmen. It is held that the death of "just anyone" will not do; the person killed in settlement of the contract must be a close kinsman. *Tahu'a* of this kind, naturally enough, are considered to be very dangerous, and very powerful. Over the course of the last generation there has been at least one violent murder in the Leeward Islands which could be laid to these beliefs. In this case a *tahu'a* was murdered by a close relative who believed that he had been made sick by the *tahu'a* and would eventually die. Probably most *tahu'a*, like Fatu, are at pains to claim that their powers come from a kinsman and involve no malevolent contracts. In describing to me some of Fatu's accomplishments several people were skeptical of his claims to have only an ancestral familiar.

Since Fatu's powers had failed, the people of the community had recourse to two other well-known *tahu'a hi'ohi'o,* who lived some distance away in other communities. Both these *tahu'a* were middle-aged men, one of them a deacon in his parish. Accounts of the cures which they had made were well known to practically every adult in the community, although the majority had never seen either of these men actually exercising his special powers. During the nine months I lived in the community there was no occasion for either of these *tahu'a* to be called in, and Fatu himself advised only one man about a sickness, in a way which did not involve communicating with his spirit familiar. For this reason I never saw a *tahu'a hi'ohi'o* in consultation with a patient, and the following account is based on the observations and testimony of others.

Fatu, whom most adults of the community had seen in action, preferred to work with a patient when only a few of the patient's closest associates and relatives were present. His procedure was to run his fingers lightly over a patient's body until he detected the precise location of the sickness by what he described as "little pecking sensations" in his fingertips. This also gave him some indication as to whether the sickness was a true sickness or a *ma'i tūpāpa'u* 'ghost sickness'. If it was decided that the patient had a ghost sickness Fatu might pronounce immediately on the cause, or else call upon his familiar to speak through his mouth, telling of what he saw. To accomplish this, Fatu would seat himself on the floor, remain quiet for a short period before going into a trancelike state associated, according to eyewitnesses, with some involuntary body movements and labored breathing. While in this state his lips moved and his *tūpāpa'u* would speak with the voice of a very old man, telling of what he saw in connection with the illness. These statements were elliptical and their meanings sometimes difficult to fathom, although the *tūpāpa'u* would answer questions from those who sought clarification of various points. After one of these sessions, which might last five minutes or so, Fatu would appear to return to consciousness very weak and exhausted, to be restored by a young couple of the community who were his usual helpers on these occasions, with massage and refreshments of coconut water or coffee. He would have no knowledge of what his familiar had said through his mouth and would be told by his helpers and others present about what had taken place. They would then work out together the meaning and implications of what had been said.

The procedures followed by other *tahu'a hi'ohi'o* are various. One from a nearby community on the same island would come only if sent for and escorted by his kinsmen who lived in the village. Instead of Fatu's light touching of the patient's body, he used limes as an aid in diagnosis. He would place a lime on a board on the ground, step on it with his full weight, and then observe the pattern made by the juice which was squashed out. Another *tahu'a hi'ohi'o* on the island had as his familiar the *tūpāpa'u* of a man who, when alive, was very fond of wine and spirits, and this man was said to expect wine to be served whenever he was called to see a patient. Both of these *tahu'a* could achieve the same trance state as Fatu had been able to, and would use it on occasion.

The most obvious occurrences of ghost sickness takes place when a foreign *tūpāpa'u* "enters into the body" of a living person, causing the person to behave in unusual and often bizarre ways. An example of this, witnessed by a number of people, had occurred in the community some years previously. A man in his thirties, whom I shall call A, was cutting copra with two companions a short distance from the village. Out of curiosity, and seeking a brief diversion from their work, they got down several old skulls from their well-known resting place in a nearby cliff. A treated one of these skulls irreverently, putting a cigarette between its teeth and laughing at it. That evening, as it got dark, he fell into violent convulsions and was incoherent and hysterical—possessed, as his companions at once knew, by the *tūpāpa'u* of the skull. Fatu was immediately sent for, and as he was paddled quickly across the bay to the patient he could, he said, see the *tūpāpa'u* of the skull moving along the shoreline in the darkness, arousing the dogs of each successive house which he passed. The *tūpāpa'u* was an old man dressed in a loincloth made of a white flour sack and he was hurrying back to the vicinity where the skull rested because he was aware that Fatu was coming to drive him away. When Fatu arrived, the patient was serene though unconscious, and was quietly restored by Fatu.

According to informants, women are generally more liable to possession by *tūpāpa'u* than men, and some women of a weak and nervous nature are particularly prone, having been possessed on several occasions. The man possessed by the *tūpāpa'u* of the skull was ordinarily of a shy and retiring disposition and had previously had no untoward experiences with ghosts. After this episode, however, both he and his wife became close associates of Fatu and used to restore him after his sessions with his familiar. For a period it was believed that he might become a *tahu'a* himself.

Visitations by a *tūpāpa'u* of the opposite sex appear to be a relatively common form of ghost sickness, and I learned of cases which had occurred in both communities. Erotic dreams are commonly described as being due to a ghost sexual partner, and are not usually spoken of as being *moemoeā* 'dreams' at all. Such experiences are generally held to be of no particular significance if they occur only infrequently and do not always involve the same ghost. Some people, though, appear to become obsessed by a particular ghost of the opposite sex, grow weak and thin, refrain from sexual intercourse with their spouses, and are given to lying around and having conversations with the *tūpāpa'u*. In such cases the *tūpāpa'u* must have driven away by a *tahu'a*. One such case involving a married woman whom I shall call B was described to me in the following terms. B had several young children at the time, and the first sign that something was wrong was when she declared herself no longer attracted to her husband and attempted to chase him from their bed at nights. She would bathe in the evenings, put on scented oil and special clothes, and lie on a separate bed, talking and laughing with a *tūpāpa'u tāne* 'male ghost'. The husband sought Fatu's help, and they went together to the house one evening when B was going through her unusual routines. Fatu and the husband sat down at a table in the room while B continued to "laugh and chatter." Fatu sat on the bed, touched her arm and asked her the meaning of what she was doing, whereupon she simply turned to face the wall and lay still. In his normal voice Fatu then commanded the *tūpāpa'u* to leave and never return. B slept soundly for the rest of the night and had no more dealings with the male ghost again. According to Fatu, the ghost was "ripped up" by his familiar.

One further example will serve to illustrate the nature of ghost sicknesses and the way in which they are diagnosed and dealt with. A man, C, on his return to the shore from his plantations one afternoon, stopped to talk with his cousin's husband, D. As they talked, he drove his long bush-knife into a nearby tree to keep it out of the way. When he reached his home he found that he had forgotten his knife and returned to the tree to retrieve it, only to find that it was no longer there. D denied all knowledge of its whereabouts, but C, convinced that he had taken it, swore at D in the stylized accepted form, wishing upon D "the wrong that D had committed on him." A month or so later, D fell sick. He would not eat, and complained of vague pains all over his body, which extensive treatment with medicines of various kinds could not remedy. Eventually, Fatu took him to live in his house. According to Fatu, one day after D had been with him a week a knife flew through the air past his head and stuck in the house thatch, just as he was stooping to go in the door. He knew then the meaning of the sickness. D readily confessed his theft of the knife. Fatu and the local deacon took him to C, to whom he made his apology, and the deacon prayed together with them both. From that time onward D began to eat more substantially, and he made a rapid recovery.

Informants described this as an instance of ghost sickness, even though no ghost had been directly involved in causing D's sickness. It was also described as a *ma'i fa'autu'a* 'retribution sickness' and some of the more pious saw the sickness and the sign of the flying knife as having been sent directly by God. I learned of numerous other incidents involving the same stylized cursing as a form of confrontation between people involved in disputes, with subsequent sicknesses and eventual reconciliations.

CONCLUSION

The account I have given of the nature of sickness and the methods of diagnosis and curing is based almost exclusively on information gathered in one relatively small rural community, and the classification of different kinds of true sicknesses represents the knowledge and practices of only one man in that community. Although he was generally acknowledged to be the best informed and most skilled of the local *tahu'a rā'au,* there were also two others in the community who were called upon to make medicines of various kinds. When their help was sought, they made their own independent diagnoses, and each of them was credited with having made successful treatments of what seemed to be minor ailments. There was no apparent rivalry between the three, and, significantly, their diagnoses of particular cases, their classifications of various true sicknesses, and the medicines which they used all differed markedly in most instances. They never consulted together on particular cases, since the accepted etiquette demanded that a patient should try the resources of one *tahu'a* at a time before moving on, if necessary, to ask another for help.

Given this range of variation in the very fundamentals of classification, diagnosis, and treatment among three semispecialists from the one small community who were, in most other matters, in close social contact with one another, it is hardly surprising that there should be considerable variations in these matters between semispecialist *tahu'a rā'au* in different rural communities and on different islands. Some indication of the range of this variation may be gathered from a comparison of the material presented here with that described by, for example, Panoff (1966) and Petard (1972). It may be accounted for by the conventions of the *tahu'a rā'au* role and by the very nature of the reality which the *tahu'a* and other participants seek to construct. For, as Fabrega has correctly pointed out, "strictly speaking, there is no object or concrete thing that is a disease, although there are tissues, hearts, livers, and respiratory passages that may demonstrate or reflect the manifestations and characteristics that we would attribute to disease" (1972, 585). There is also some variation between Levy's (1973) and my accounts of the Tahitian concepts of *vārua* and *tūpāpa'u* and of the nature and derivation of the powers attributed to various kinds of *tahu'a*. But these are, on the whole, minor, and relate less to "nuclear beliefs" than to the more "ancillary" ones where there is scope for individual speculation and elaboration of the "furniture of the other world" (Firth 1948, 27).

It would, I think, be wrong to see these variations as due to the beliefs, classifications, prescriptions, and so forth being but decadent, imperfect remnants of what was once a more coherent, unified body of beliefs and practices. In his authoritative account of late eighteenth and early nineteenth century Tahitian culture, Oliver observes that:

> among those who dealt with human ailments there was wide variation both in fundamental approach and in procedural detail. Some specialists acted primarily as priests, others as shamans, others as magicians, and still others as physicians or surgeons or bone setters, with only slight dependence on spirit aid. Moreover, within each of these "specialties" there had developed individualized techniques and skills, and there were probably many practitioners who combined, in varying proportions, the elements of several specialties. It is more than likely that in addition to the presence of such specialists in this society, every man and woman was something of a practitioner himself, with his own little stock of remedies and skills. (1974, 476)

The priests, shamans, and other specialists of Oliver's account have long since disappeared from Tahitian life, along with much of the rest of the complex traditional Polynesian culture which he describes. But although Tahitian curing practices might have been transformed over two centuries of intensive European contact, there are also some striking continuities of both ideology and technique. The "vulnerary herbs" which Banks mentioned are still used, and Tahitians still maintain, as they did to Brodie, a preference for them over "European physic." The procedures followed by Pearse's "native sorcerer or diviner" are in essence strikingly similar to those which are still practiced today. These continuities are probably not due entirely to the efficacy of the medicines as this would be construed in western pharmacological terms, or even to the so-called psychosomatic nature of the ghost sicknesses and their stylized cures. Like other medical systems, Tahitian medicine is involved with considerably more than curing in these terms. It is based on distinctive ideas about the fundamental nature and meaning of sickness and a particular context and style of social relationships.

In my view, all instances of *ma'i tūpāpa'u*, and not only those which might be labeled by Tahitians as *ma'i fa'autua* 'retribution sickness', involve an element of social conflict or other disturbances of the moral order. In the case of the stolen knife the element of conflict is clear, and was brought into public view by the very process of treatment. The man possessed by the ghost of the skull which he had mistreated had behaved in a sacrilegious manner in a semipublic situation, and given the Tahitian views about how human remains should be treated he might well have expected some sort of punishment for his foolhardiness. The case of the male ghost is somewhat less clear, since I did not learn anything of the personal relationship between the woman and her husband prior to her involvement with the *tūpāpa'u*. When I knew them there was nothing in their calm, apparently placid relationship which called for comment of any kind from others in the community, and I neglected to pursue the matter any further. I would be surprised, however, if their relationship had been entirely serene prior to the incident.

Although the moral element is most evident in instances of ghost sickness, it is also not entirely absent from Tahitian views of their other categories of sickness. Although *ma'i mau* 'true sickness' may sometimes just happen for unknown reasons, freedom from sicknesses of any kind can be held up as a sign of virtue and a blameless life. This was brought out by several informants, always in relation to themselves or their families, when discussing the misfortunes of others. The same ideas are clearly expressed about those instances of *ma'i* which I have classed together as injuries. Injuries, like true sicknesses, may at times just happen, but under some circumstances are held to be virtually certain to occur. Tahitians maintain that fishing on the Sabbath or any other holy day renders one liable to attack by sharks or other fish—"even quite small ones" which usually flee at the sight of humans. Similar injuries are likely to happen to men who go to sea after a domestic quarrel which has not been made up.

The proposition that sickness of any kind may well be a punishment has a clear latent function in the field of social control. But it also has more subtle implications which go beyond the possibility that some people may be simply deterred from wrongdoing by their fear that they might get sick as a consequence. One of the striking features of rural Tahitian life is the manner in which people gossip about the indispositions of others. News of this sort travels rapidly through the usual networks and through casual encounters, characteristically accompanied by laconic comment and discussion of possible causes. For example, a man fell from his bicycle one day, injuring his wrist, and the news of this came to be spread with the embellishment that it only served him right for having beaten his daughter unjustly several days previously. Again, a woman died with dramatic suddenness from an internal hemorrhage, and in the many ensuing discussions about this there was a general consensus that her death was a punishment on her husband for laziness; she had done much of the work of the household, which he would now have to undertake himself. And the tragedy in which an interisland launch swamped, drowning a number of the party of Mormon converts on board, was universally acknowledged to be a punishment, albeit a rather drastic one, for their abandoning the Protestant faith.

It is apparent that this constant moral commentary on *ma'i* of all kinds taps a whole hidden vein of local conflicts, tensions, and rivalries, and that it can serve to crystallize and provide a focus for public opinion about the sick person and his or her associates. If the sickness should then warrant consultation with a *tahu'a hi'ohi'o* there is a ready-made consensus of opinion and approbation which he may, if he chooses, draw upon in making a diagnosis. The process of diagnosis and treatment is thus a means of mobilizing the consensus and putting it into effect to redress some moral wrong. If this is so, the question arises as to why the process of effectively sanctioning public opinion should be so apparently haphazard (depending on sickness to focus attention on the issues) and so laboriously indirect and circuitous. I do not wish to suggest that Tahitians do not settle local differences and disputes by other more direct and straightforward means, but it is nevertheless true that there is no office or group in the rural communities which has the authority to arbitrate disputes and resolve deep-seated differences.

The conversion of the Tahitians by the London Missionary Society missionaries in the earlier part of the nineteenth century and the subsequent annexation of the islands by France brought about the downfall of the indigenous authority system, which in the rural areas has never been effectively replaced. The introduction of French law provided a framework for Tahitian society to develop according to a European model of individual tenure and small peasant holdings, but Tahitians have generally chosen instead to hold their land rights in common, transmitting them by the cognatic French laws of succession. Rural economic life involves intricate strategies of cooperation and compromise among bodies of co-owners, for whom the law provides no really clear-cut organizational structure. The rural communities, made up basically of people who have simply inherited land rights in the vicinity, are de facto entities, neither traditionally Polynesian in organization nor French, and lack a stable, clear-cut, and explicit authority structure. Local government is minimal and largely ineffectual.

Within these communities social relationships are egalitarian and intensely multiplex in nature. Individuals are bound to one another by relations based on propinquity, religious associations, land ownership (and its associated economic enterprises), kinship, marriage, friendship, sex, and broad age divisions; and, most importantly, these relations are always with the same relatively restricted set of other people. Factions, cliques, and shifting coalitions are evident in all local affairs, coloring nearly all social relationships. In my view, these facts are related to some of the distinctive qualities of Tahitian interaction, which have been noticed and commented on by numerous writers. Given the relatively fluid unformalized role structure and the multiplex character of community relationships, interactions have a tentative, cautious aspect, as though highly attuned to the complex social implications of every move. A gentle, subtle indirection is far more appropriate to Tahitian social style and sensitivities than open confrontations or direct persuasion.[5]

Seen in this context, Tahitian doctrines about sickness and curing take on an added dimension. Not only do they provide a set of explanatory principles for sickness itself and a device for social control and the delivery of psychological support for those who are sick. They also play a part in maintaining the morality of social relationships within Tahitian communities, by invoking the authority of both the Christian God and Polynesian spirits to pronounce indirectly the judgment of neighbors and peers. This aspect of Tahitian healing may even be partly recognized by Tahitians themselves, who commonly maintain that ghost sicknesses are essentially *Tahitian* sicknesses, to which Europeans (who are rarely involved and implicated in the intimate tangle of community affairs in the same way as Tahitians) are expected to be immune.[6]

NOTES

1. Two periods of field research, of eighteen months and two months, were sponsored by the U. S. National Institute of Mental Health and the University of Auckland, respectively. An earlier version of this paper was presented at an Anthropology Department seminar at the Research School of Pacific Studies, Canberra, in January 1975 and I am most grateful to Dr. John B. Haviland for the helpful comments which he made on that version. I am also grateful to Professor Ralph Bulmer of Auckland University for his useful criticisms of an earlier draft.

2. Lemaitre 1973. Lemaitre's information, gathered mainly I think on Tahiti, is completely independent of my own.

3. I had thought this to be an original observation, but Nigel Baumber has since drawn my attention to Hocart's statement (1929, 62) about Lau medicines: "Diseases are not diagnosed by symptoms but by the cure that happens to succeed."

4. Hi'ohi'o is the reduplicative of hi'o 'to look, examine' and ta'ata hi'ohi'o is a "clairvoyant."

5. A number of these ideas are set out in more detail in Hooper 1975.

6. The only exception to this is the ghost sickness which is believed to affect any person who violates the site of a Tahitian *marae*.

APPENDIX

This appendix contains the recipes of medicines for various *ma'i mau* 'true sicknesses' known to one *tahu'a rā'au*, who dictated them to me on various occasions over a period of several weeks. The varieties of true sickness distinguished are his own, and they are given here in the order in which he gave them, together with his brief remarks on the relevant symptoms. I have attempted to follow closely the order and style of his presentation and the result is in fact close to the sort of written record which is made by Tahitians when they commit recipes to personal and family notebooks. This man did not, however, have his own written record of recipes and worked entirely from memory. He repeated several complex recipes for me in exactly the same form that he had given up to ten days previously.

As the term *rā'au* implies, most of the ingredients used are plant material, but two of them included in the glossary below are common echinoderms. I have used local names in the recipes, as they were used by the *tahu'a* and commonly understood by others in the Iles sous-le-vent. As with fish names, these occasionally differ from those commonly used in Tahiti. Through the kindness and interest of Mme. Aurora Natua of the Papeete Museum I was able to record many of these differences, which are noted in the glossary below. I collected specimens of many of the plants used, which have been identified by Dr. A. Orchard, botanist at the Auckland War Memorial Museum. I am most grateful to Dr. Orchard for his help. The ingredients marked in the glossary with an asterisk were made by him and are deposited at the Museum. Notes on the other identifications are given in the glossary.

GLOSSARY OF INGREDIENT NAMES

ʻaʻeho	*Erianthus floridulus* (Schut. Mant) acc. to Nadeaud 1873.
ʻaero fai	*Achyranthes aspera L.
ahi	*Santalum insulare* (Bertero Mss.) acc. to Nadeaud 1873.
ʻahiʻa	*Eugenia malaccensis* acc. to Chabouis n.d. Vol. I.
ʻahiʻa ʻavaʻava	*Oxalis corniculata L. According to Mme. Natua, this is known in Tahiti as *patoa ʻavaʻava*.
ʻaito haʻari	*Psilotum nudum (L.) Palisot.
ʻānani tahiti	*Citrus* spp.
ʻape	*Alocasia macrorrhiza* L. acc. to Barrau 1961 and Papy 1954.
ʻati	*Calophyllum inophyllum* L.
ʻaua	*Terminalia cattapa L. = *T. glabrata* Forst. According to both local informants and Mme. Natua, this is known as *ʻautaraʻa* in Tahiti.
ʻaute	*Broussonetia papyrifera (L.) Vent.
ʻaute ʻuʻumu	*Hibiscus rosa-sinensis L.
au fenua	A river slime.
fara	*Pandanus* spp.
feʻe	*Ophiocoma scolopendrina* Lmk. acc. to Chabouis n.d., vol. 2. Known in Tahiti as *maʻamaʻatai* according to Mme. Natua.
hoi	*Dioscorea bulbifera* L. acc. to Barrau 1961 and Papy 1954.
mape	*Inocarpus edulis* Forster acc. to Barrau 1961.
mataʻura	*Cyathula prostrata Blume. According to informants this is known in Tahiti as *toroʻura*.
mati	*Ficus tinctoria* Forst. acc. to Nadeaud 1873 and Papy 1954.
matie	*Echinochloa colonum (?)
meiʻa	*Musa* spp.
metuapuaʻa	*Polypodium nigrescens* Bl. acc. to Lemaitre 1973.
miro	*Thespesia populnea* (D.C.) acc. to Nadeaud 1873.
moahauʻaino	*Cardamine sarmentosa Forst. In Tahiti, according to Mme. Natua, this is known as *pātoapurahi*.
moemoe	*Phyllanthus nirari L.
mōʻu upoʻo hina	*Kyllinga monocephela Rottb. According to Mme. Natua, this is known in Tahiti as *matie upoʻo ʻuoʻuo*.
niu	*Leucas flaccida R. Br. According to local informants, this is known as *niuhiti* in Tahiti.

nono	*Morinda citrifolia* L. acc. to Barrau 1961.
'ofe'ofe	**Centotheca lappacea* (L.) Desv.
pāpati	*Ipomea spp. Informants said that this name was not known in Tahiti.
pia or *pia mutu*	*Tacca leontopetaloides* (L.) Kuntze (*T. pinnatifida* Forster) acc. to Barrau 1961.
piri'ate	**Vandellia crustacea* Benth. According to both Mme. Natua and local informants, this plant is known as *ha'eha'a* in Tahiti.
piripapa	**Portulacca oleracea*. This may be known in Tahiti as *'aturi*.
piripiri	**Cenchrus echinatus* L.
pito	**Ophioglossum reticulatum* L. According to Mme. Natua, this is known as *ti'apito* in Tahiti.
pitorea	**Polygonum glabrum* Willd. Known in Tahiti as *tamore*, acc. to Mme. Natua.
pua'a veoveo	**Crateva religiosa* Forst.
pūrau	*Hibiscus tileaceous* acc. to Chabouis n.d., vol. 1.
ta'ata'ahiara	*Dichrocephala latifolia* acc. to Nadeaud 1873.
taino'a	**Cassytha filiformis* L.
ti'a'iri	*Aleurites moluccana* Wildenow (*A.triloba* J. R. and G. Forster) acc. to Barrau 1961.
tiare tahiti	*Gardenia tahitiensis* acc. to Chabouis n.d., vol. 1.
titi	*Davallia solida (Forst.) SW. Known in Tahiti as *ti'ati-'amoua*.
tō patu	*tō* is *Saccharum officinarum* L. acc. to Barrau 1961. *Patu* refers to a variety which is distinguished.
tōhetupou	*Geophila repens (L.) I. M. Johnston = *G. herbacea* etc.?
toro'e'a	**Canthium barbatum* (Forst.) Seem. In Tahiti, according to Mme. Natua, this is known as *torotea*.
tou	*Cordia subcordata* Lamarck acc. to Barrau 1961.
tuava	*Psidium guajava* L. acc. to Barrau 1961.
'uru	*Artocarpus altilis* (Parkinson) Fosberg. acc. to Barrau 1961.
vai'anu	**Adenostemma lavenia* (L.) Kuntze = *A. viscosum*.
vana	An Echinoderm. *Hechinoxtrix* (?) acc. to Chabouis n.d., vol. 2.
vī 'ohurepi'o	*Mangifera indica L. *'Ohurepi'o* is a variety name.

MEDICINES

Ira

1. *Ira miti* — Found characteristically in children, who feel sick and have a fever at 10 A.M. and feel better at 2 P.M.; *miti* in Tahitian means "sea water" and there is held to be a connection between the symptoms and the diurnal movements of the tide.

   40 fresh leaves of *tiare tahiti*
   40 fresh leaves of *'aute*
   The water of one "black" coconut

   Pound the leaves with a stone, wrap in a cloth, and pour the coconut water through it. Boil the wrapped leaves in the coconut water. Bathe the whole body of the child in the liquid and also give it two soupspoonsful to drink.

2. *Ira vaeha'a* — A pain on one side of the face only, which may occur in both children and adults.

   Ingredients used are the same as those for *Ira miti*.

   If the pain affects the right side of the face then use only the the right side of the leaves; if the left side of the face, then only the left side of the leaves. When the medicine is made, divide it equally between two bowls. Heat two fist-sized stones in an earth-oven until very hot, and drop them into a bowl. Cover the patient's head with a sheet and have him breathe the steam and vapors as an inhalation. Then use the other half of the medicine. Some may also be drunk.

3. *Ira 'āhure* — Inflammation and breaking of the skin around the urethra of female children.

   1 handful of red *taino'a*
   1 handful of white *taino'a*
   1 handful of *piri'ate*
   1 handful of *pāpati*
   4 drinking coconuts

   Pound the plant matter to a pulp and divide it into two equal portions. Wrap each portion in a piece of cloth, and using the water of two coconuts for each portion, wring the juices from the portion into the coconut water. Use one portion of the medicine (consisting of the coconut water and expressed juices) to bathe the affected part; if possible, have the patient sit in it. The other portion should be drunk.

4. *Ira tui* — A discharge of puss and matter from the ears, and a lot of matter in the eyes.

   30 fresh leaves of *tiare tahiti*
   30 leaves of *'aute 'u'umu*

1 handful of *niu*
1 handful of *vai'anu*
1 handful of *mata'ura*
1 handful of *moemoe*
1 handful of *moahau'a'ino*
2 red leaves of *mape*
2 black leaves of *mape*
1 handful of leaves of *vī 'ava'ava* (a kind of vī)

Pound these ingredients to a pulp and wrap in a cloth. Express the juices into the water of six green drinking coconuts, and heat. The eyes and ears should be bathed with the medicine, and some given to the patient to drink.

5. *Ira 'ute*

Red, painful lips of children.

3 opened flowers of *tiare tahiti*
3 terminal shoots of *tiare tahiti*
30 terminal shoots of *'aute*
1 coffee bowl of fresh water

Pound the ingredients to a pulp, wrap in a cloth, and express the juices into the water. Bathe the lips and give some of the medicine to be drunk, adding a little sugar.

6. *Ira nīnamu*

Occurs only in children, the symptoms being dark lips and eyes, fever, headache, and desire for sleep.

2 handfuls of leaves of *tiati'a mou'a*
2 handfuls of leaves of *toro'e'a*
1 banana leaf, of the variety known as *meia 'ore'a*. Only the stalk of the leaf is used.
1 young shoot of the variety of pandanus known as *pae'ore*. Discard the stalk, taking only the leaf part.
1 branch of *fara nīnamu*, as long as a forearm. Discard the outside bark, taking only the inside bark to be scraped into the medicine.

Pound the ingredients to a pulp, wrap in a cloth, and express the juices into the water of four drinking coconuts. Boil, and while it is still hot, sprinkle it with the fingers over the whole body. Two teaspoons may be given to drink, three times daily.

7. *Ira hitirere*

Known also as *Ira hui*. Startling in young children.

The same medicine is used as for *Ira nīnamu*.

8. *Hua ira*

A swelling of a child's penis, associated with inflammation, and, sometimes, a black color.

12 opened flowers of *tiare tahiti*
1 handful of *piripiri totetō* (a kind of piripiri)
1 section of *tō tore* (a kind of to)

Tahitian Healing

Crush the *tō* to a pulp. Crush the other ingredients to a pulp separately. Mix the pulps, wrap in a cloth, and express the juices. Give to the patient to drink.

Another medicine for the same sickness is as follows:

1 handful of *pito*
1 handful of *piri'ate*
1 handful of *vai'anu*
1 handful of *mata'ura*
1 handful of *niu*

Pound the ingredients to a pulp, wrap in a cloth, and express the juices into the water of three black drinking coconuts. Boil, and bathe the affected parts, also giving some of the medicine to be drunk.

Māriri

1. *Māriri 'otu'i ate* Symptoms are a fever and a pain *inside* any part of the trunk of the body—not in any part of the leg or on the outside of the body. The patient characteristically wants to drink a lot of water.

    1 handful of flower buds of *matie*
    1 handful of flower buds of *piripiri*
    1 handful of flower buds of *'ofe'ofe*
    1 kernel of a sprouting coconut

    Pound the ingredients to a pulp, wrap in a cloth, and express the juices into the water of one "black" drinking coconut. To be given to the patient to drink. Then take the "dross" from which the juice has been expressed, dampen it, and bind it as a poultice over the painful region.

2. *Māriri fati* Fever, with periods of chills, and a continual cough.

    4 pieces, about 4 inches long, of *titi*
    4 pieces, about 4 inches long, of *metua pua'a*
    4 terminal shoots of *tiare tahiti*
    4 flower buds of *ta'ata'ahiara*
    1 handful of flower buds of *'ofe'ofe*
    1 handful of flower buds of *mōupo'ohina*

    Pound the ingredients to a pulp, wrap, and express juices into a liter of fresh water, adding some sugar. Give some to drink, and also bathe the whole body with it. Massage is also helpful while body is bathed.

3. *Māriri 'ai ta'ata* A swelling which has no matter in it, which may appear both inside and outside the body. For one inside the body, there is no medicine—but there is one for the outside. The informant identified this as cancer. For external application, the following medicine is used.

2 roots of *pia mutu*
1 red tuber of wild *hoi*
1 white tuber of wild *hoi*
1 handful of both the leaves and vine of *pāpati*

Pound these ingredients together, adding no water, and wrap in a cloth. Bind some of the pounded matter onto the swollen region.

The following medicine is given to be drunk.

A piece, four fingerwidths square, of the bark of *ti'a'iri*
The water of one "black" drinking coconut
1 handful of the white roots of *pūrau* which can be found in water beside a *pūrau* tree

Pound the roots and bark, wrap, and express juices into the coconut water. Put the medicine back into the coconut and leave it for a while. This may be rubbed on the body and also drunk—one lot of medicine per day.

4. *Māriri fefera* A red mottled color appearing over the whole body, associated with fever. The informant suggested that it is Rubella.

2 tubers of *nūmera*

Pound to a pulp, wrap, and express juice into water of one "black" coconut. Give to drink and bathe the body with it.

5. *Māriri 'ere'ere* This sickness has no symptoms more specific than high fever, pain all over the body, and thirst. If it is fatal, the body turns black after death.

10 green fruits of *vī 'ohurepi'o*. Cut off the skin and grate the fruits onto a plate.
8 pieces of *titi* 4 inches long
8 pieces of *metua pua'a,* 4 inches long
8 opened flowers of *tiare tahiti*
40 terminal shoots of *tiare tahiti*
40 leaves of *'aua*. Discard the leafy parts, taking only the stalks.
40 leaves of *'ahi'a*
1 handful of *pito*
1 handful of *piri'ate*
8 flower buds of *ta'ata'ahiara*

Pound these ingredients together and mix in the grated *vī*. Wrap and express the juice into the water of forty *omoto* drinking coconuts to which has been added one kilo of brown sugar, and the juice of eight limes *(taporo)*. Pour the whole mixture into a demijohn and use it to bathe the patient and for the patient to drink.

6. *Māriri pu'upu'u* Pimples on the surface of the body and legs, which have no matter in them.

The kernels of 4 *opa'a* coconuts, grated
1 piece, four fingerwidths square, of the bark of *'ati*
1 piece, four fingerwidths square, of the bark of *'ahi'a mā'ohi*
1 piece, four fingerwidths square, of the bark of *tou*
1 piece, four fingerwidths square, of the bark of *miro*
1 piece, four fingerwidths square, of the bark of *vī 'ava'ava*
5 plants of *mō'u upo'o hina*

Express the milk from the grated coconut and put the *mō'u upo'o hina* into it. Put in a frying pan and cook slowly, adding two teaspoonsful (one at a time) of *pia* (the flour made from *pia mutu*). When it is cooked, put about two inches of the liquid into a glass to be drunk. It has a very laxative effect. The remainder of the medicine may be spread on the affected parts. Patient should not drink cold water, only warm water or coconut water.

7. *Hua māriri*

A red swelling of the male genitalia.

20 leaves of *'aua*
20 terminal shoots of *tiare tahiti*
1 handful of *piripiri*
1 handful of *matie*

Pound these ingredients together to a pulp, wrap, and express the juices into the water of six "black" drinking coconuts. This may be poured or sprinkled on the genitals three times daily.

8. *Māriri pūfe-'efe'e*

A redness and swelling of either or both arms and legs. The redness not confined to one spot but spread over the whole limb. It is associated with pain and fever. *Fe'efe'e* is the Tahitian term for elephantiasis and this sickness is probably filarial.

1 six-inch square of the bark of *tou*
1 six-inch square of the bark of a "black" coconut
1 six-inch square of the bark of *miro*
1 six-inch square of the bark of *pūrau*

All these should be crushed together as much as possible, then water added and the mixture sprinkled on the affected limb(s).

A drinking medicine for this same sickness uses all the above ingredients, but of the size of four square inches and the addition of the following:

1 handful of flower buds of *piripiri*
1 handful of flower buds of *matie*
20 terminal shoots of *tiare tahiti*

All these should be pounded together and the juices extracted by pressing into the water of one "black" coconut. Add a gallon of water. Add sugar. Drink.

Another medicine is as follows:

2 mature fruits of *nono*
2 immature fruits of *nono*
2 mature leaves of *nono*
2 immature leaves of *nono*
1 handful of *mataʻura*

Pound together to a pulp. Add no water, but spread the pulp on the affected limb.

Yet another treatment is to wet a cloth with the medicine for *Māriri ʻereʻere* and press it on the limb.

Tui

1. *Tui hotete*   A swelling, or swellings, on the lower jaw and throat and below the ears on the side of the neck. The swellings have matter in them.

2 fully mature leaves of *nono*
2 immature leaves of *nono*
2 leaves of *ʻaute*

Pound these ingredients to a pulp and express the juices into the water of one mature coconut into which the kernel has been grated. Heat this liquid with a hot stone, cover it with a cloth, and when it is cold give it to be drunk all at once. If the swelling should break, scorch a leaf of *tafaie* on a fire, spread *monoi* 'scented coconut oil' on it, and put on the broken head of the swelling.

2. *Papā tui*   A swelling, inside only of the neck region. No matter in the swelling and it is highly infectious. "If one child gets it, all children get it."

5 opened flowers of *tiare tahiti*
The inside bark of one stalk of *nono*

Pound these ingredients into a pulp, wrap, and express the juices into water. Mix into this water a kind of store-bought soap known as *puʻa nātura,* stirring it until it becomes thick and hard. The stirring should be done in *one* direction only (either clockwise or counterclockwise) with no reversal. Spread over the neck.

3. *Tui houhou*   Little pimples over the body and scalp, with matter in them.

1 handful of flower buds of *niu*
1 handful of leaves and flower buds of *mataʻura*
1 handful of *tiʻapito*
1 handful of *piriʻate*
3 terminal shoots of *tiare atatea*

1 inch of the tuber of a *nūmera*
3 sections of *tō patu* (a variety called *tō piavere* in Tahiti)

Pound the *tō* to a pulp. Pound the other ingredients together into a pulp and mix with the *tō* pulp. This juice is to be drunk three times daily.

4. *Tui he'a* Yellow fluid and matter discharging from the ears.

3 seeds of *ti'a'iri*. Discard the skin and take only the kernel.
1 handful of *pito*
1 handful of *piri'ate*
1 small branch of *tiare tahiti*
1 small branch of *pua'a veoveo*
3 mature leaves of *tou*
3 immature leaves of *tou*
Fruit of *mati*

Take the *tou* leaves and express the juice from *mati* fruit onto them until they are thoroughly wet. Pound, wrap, and put to one side. Scrape the inside bark from the *tiare tahiti* and *pua'a veoveo* branches and pulp them together with the other ingredients. Crush some *tō* to get about one liter of juice. Express the juice from the two lots of pulp to this juice and give it to be drunk.

5. *Tui topa i roto i te 'ōuma* This is a *tui,* a swelling from the head which has fallen inside the body.

7 leaves of *vī 'ava'ava*
7 flower buds of *niu*
2 fruits of *miro,* one mature and the other immature. Use only the kernels, discarding the skins.

Pound these ingredients together, wrap, and express the juice into a little fresh water. Grate a pinch of *'ahi* wood into the mixture and add a level teaspoonful of brown sugar. Stir, and give to be drunk. Some may be massaged onto the chest.

6. *Tui 'ai roro* Symptoms are matter from the nose and in the eyes, and headache. Most frequently in children. If not treated it forms a "bag" on the side of the brain—according to the informant, like cancer.

2 mature leaves of *tou*
2 immature leaves of *tou*
2 terminal shoots of *tiare tahiti*
2 opened flowers of *tiare tahiti*
4 flower buds of *'aute,* taking only the central parts of the buds

Pound these ingredients to a pulp, wrap. Take one coffee bowl of fresh water and add to it one level teaspoon of brown sugar. Express the juices into this water and divide the resultant mixture in half. One half to be drunk, a soupspoonful at a time; the other to be bathed on the head.

He'a

1. He'a pa'a

Dry, cracked lips; may affect both children and adults.

3 plants of *piri'ate 'ōtāne* (*'ōtāne* is the term for male plants and animals, and the *'ōtāne* in this case is red in color)
3 plants of *piri'ate 'ōvahine* (*'ōvahine* is the female, in this case white in color)
12 plants of *ti'apito 'ōtāne* (the *'ōtāne* in this case is the one which flowers)
2 sections of *tō*

Pound these ingredients to a pulp, wrap, and express juices into a bowl. To be drunk only, not bathed on the lips. The patient should then be purged.

2. He'a ha'amae

Occurs only in children, who are thin and don't eat well, having appetite for only charred foods or raw food like banana.

1 large bundle of *ti'apito*
1 large bundle of *piri'ate*
4 mature leaves of *tou*
4 immature leaves of *tou*
1 section, four fingerwidths square, of bark of *tou*
1 handful of leaves of *autara'a mou'a*. Discard the leafy parts, taking only the leaf stalks.
4 "pimpled, rough" leaves of *ahi'a*
4 smooth leaves of *ahi'a*
2 flower buds of *fara*. Use only the inside portions.
2 young *'ā'eho*, at the stage where it just appears above ground, with two leaves only
Fruit of *mati*

Express the juice from *mati* fruit over the leaves of *tou* until they are well wetted. Pound the leaves to a pulp, together with the other ingredients. Wrap, and express the juices into the water of four "black" drinking coconuts. Put about a soupspoonful of *au fenua* into the mixture. Stir and drink. When well made, this medicine froths a lot.

A second medicine for this same sickness is as follows:

8 mature leaves of *tou*
8 immature leaves of *tou*

Tahitian Healing

12 opened flowers of *tiare tahiti*. (If there are no flowers, then the terminal shoots will do.)
Fruit of *mati*

Express the *mati* juice onto the *tou* leaves and when they are wet pound the leaves and other ingredients together into a pulp. Wrap, and express the juice into a gallon of water until it is red in color. Add a half-kilo of brown sugar. To be bathed on the body and also drunk.

3. He'a tupito A pain in the navel and the surrounding region, especially when eating. Occurs in both children and adults.

4 flower buds of *'uru pae'a* (a variety of *'uru*)
2 flower buds of *tō patu*
4 sections of *tō*

Pound the *tō* until pulpy. Pound the other ingredients and add to the *tō*. Wrap, and express juices into a bowl. Some to be poured into the navel three times daily and some to be drunk.

A second medicine for this is as follows:

4 flower buds of *'uru pae'a*
4 sections of *tō*

Pound the *tō*. Pound the buds and add to the *tō* juice. Some to be poured into the navel three times daily and the rest drunk.

The following is a third medicine:

1 basketful *('o'ini)* of *pito*
1 basketful *('o'ini)* of *piri'ate*

Pound to a pulp, wrap, and express juices into a gallon of *tō* juice. To be drunk only.

4. He'a tupē Small, very itchy pimples on body, face, and legs.

3 black *'ina* (sea urchins)
3 white *'ina* (sea urchins)
3 red *fe'e*
3 black *fe'e*
1 handful of *pito*
1 handful of *piri'ate*
1 coffee bowl of fruit of *tōhetupou*
4 *opa'a* coconuts
5 *mō'u upo'o hina*

> Cut the coconuts, saving the water from only one of them. Grate the four coconuts into the *mō'u upo'o hina*. Pound the other ingredients into a pulp, wrap, and express juices into the *mō'u upo'o hina*. Add one handful of corn starch (available at local store) and stir. Boil this all in some water and add one soupspoon of sugar. About one inch of this mixture to be drunk and the rest to be put aside in a bottle for annointing on the body.

'Ōpī

There is only one variety of this sickness. According to the informant it is not indigenous to Tahiti, but was brought by the Chinese. Urination is very painful, and there is matter and blood in the urine, which smells badly.

> 20 seeds of *ti'a'iri*
> 20 terminal shoots of *tiare tahiti*
>
> Pound together to a pulp, wrap, and express the juices into the water of one "black" coconut. The patient should drink it all and will be cured unless the sickness is very severe.

Tona

Only one variety of this sickness as well. Symptoms are sores on the penis, with matter in them, and open sores around the mouth. The eyebrows fall out. The informant maintains that European doctors now have a good cure for this sickness, though in former days they did not.

> 1 four-fingerwidth square of the bark of *'ati*
> 1 four-fingerwidth square of the bark of *tou*
> 1 four-fingerwidth square of the bark of *miro*
> 1 four-fingerwidth square of the bark of *vī 'ava'ava*
> 1 four-fingerwidth square of the bark of *'ānani tahiti*
> 1 four-fingerwidth square of the bark of *'ahi'a*
> 1 four-fingerwidth square of the bark of *tiare tahiti*
> 5 plants of *mō'u upo'o hina*
>
> Grate four mature coconuts and place the five *mō'u upo'o hina* in it. Pound the other ingredients as much as possible and add them to the gratings and cook with a handful of corn starch from the store. Drink two inches of the oily liquid in a glass, and leave the rest to be rubbed on affected parts. The patient should be told to bathe his sores in sea water out on the barrier reef.

'O

1. *'O fāura* — Swellings which "creep" down from inside the anus. Are itchy and "eat" the anus. The several "eyes" of the swellings should be pricked with a needle to release blood so that the swellings collapse. There are two medicines, one for application and the other for drinking.

1 plant of *moa hauʻaʻino*

Pound the plant to a pulp. Squeeze the juice from part of the pulp onto the anus. The remaining pulp should be bound by cloths onto the anus.

1 plant of *moahauʻaʻino*
3 opened flowers of *tiare tahiti*
2 terminal shoots of *tiare tahiti*
3 pieces of young root of "black" coconut
3 pieces of young root of "red" coconut
3 pieces, about 4 inches long, of *titi*
3 pieces, about 4 inches long, of *metua puaʻa*

Pound these ingredients to a pulp, wrap, and express the juices into about two inches of water in a bowl. To be drunk three times daily until used up.

2. ʻO ʻuaʻa

The same sickness as ʻO *fāura* but one which has progressed to a further stage. If not treated, the patient dies, eaten from the anus up into the interior. It cannot be cured by lancing or cutting out.

3 plants of *moahauʻaʻino*
3 plants of *piriʻate*

Pound to a pulp and add *monoi* 'scented coconut oil'. Squeeze onto the swellings.

3. ʻO ʻamu

Swellings inside the lower bowel which do not appear outside. May also grow in other parts of inside of body.

2 fully mature fruits of *nono*
2 fruits from a *nono* which also has flowers on it
2 plants of *moahauʻaʻino*
2 small roots, 2 inches long, of "black" coconut
2 small roots, 2 inches long, of "red" coconut
2 terminal shoots of *tiare tahiti*

Pound these ingredients together into a pulp. Squeeze the juices from the pulp onto the anus and if possible pour some into the rectum. Some juice may also be drunk.

A drinking medicine for the same complaint is as follows:

1 piece, four fingerwidths square, of bark of *tou*
12 pieces, 4 inches long, of *metua puaʻa*
Fruit of *mati*

Express the *mati* juice onto the *tou* bark until it is thoroughly wet. Pound the bark until a pulp. Pound the *metua puaʻa* to a pulp. Express the juices from both pulps into a bowl, add a teaspoon of sugar, and then drink this liquid.

4. *'O pararī*   A sickness found only in women who have given birth, and especially when they are old. The patient coughs a great deal.

8 pieces, 4 inches long, of *titi*
8 pieces, 4 inches long, of *metua pua'a*
8 terminal shoots of *tiare tahiti*
1 handful of *moahau'a'ino*
1 handful of *'ofe'ofe*
1 handful of flower buds of *tuava*
1 handful of *'aito ha'ari*

Pound the ingredients to a pulp, wrap, and express the juices into two handfuls of fresh water. Divide this into three parts and drink one part at a time over the course of the day.

Another treatment for this sickness is to take two handfuls of flower buds of *tuava* and heat them in a pan of water. The patient should sit with her feet in the water and with her legs and thighs covered by a cloth, so that the steam goes up between her legs.

5. *'O fati*   This kind of *'o* is caused by an old broken bone which has "come back" to give trouble. The patient coughs a great deal.

4 pieces, 4 inches long, of *titi*
4 pieces, 4 inches long, of *metua pua'a*
4 roots, 4 inches long, of "black" coconut
4 roots, 4 inches long, of "red" coconut
4 terminal shoots of *tiare tahiti*
1 handful of *moahau'a'ino*

Pound to a pulp, wrap, and express juices into two inches of fresh water in a bowl. Add no sugar. Should be drunk three times.

6. *'O 'oūma*   Pain in the chest and constant coughing.

The soft kernel of 1 "black" coconut at the stage known as *'ōuo*
1 handful of *moahau'a'ino*
1 handful of *piri'ate*
1 handful of flower buds of *ta'ata'ahiara*
8 pieces of *tō*, about 6 inches long

Pound the *tō* to a pulp, then add the pulped other ingredients. To be drunk in three sessions.

10
Midwives and Midwifery in Western Samoa

Patricia J. Kinloch

Western Samoa is a group of islands located in the Polynesian triangle of the Pacific Ocean. It is a group of high islands situated approximately 15 degrees south of the equator. There are four islands, each covered with tropical forest. The two large islands, Upolu and Savai'i, each have a road which circles the island. Upolu also has two roads which cross the interior. The roads in Upolu are good enough to allow easy access to Apia, the capital. The roads on Savai'i are not as good. There are no roads on the two smaller islands, Manono and Apolima. Savai'i and Upolu are linked by a ferry service which runs several times a day. There is also an air link between the two larger islands. Telephone communication is possible from some parts of Savai'i and Upolu to the Apia urban area.

The people reside in villages located along the shoreline of the different islands. The roads run through the middle of most of the villages. Where this has not happened, whole villages have sometimes moved from their original location to one beside the road.

The population of the independent nation of Western Samoa was almost 152,000 in 1976. Nearly two-thirds of the population (92,798, or 61 percent) were under twenty years of age, while less than one-twentieth (6,912, or 4.5 percent) were over sixty years of age (Dept. of Statistics 1979, Table 1). Meleiseā (1979, 267–68) notes that

> missionary teaching and official programmes promoting maternal and infant welfare have now resulted in a state of incipient overpopulation in Western Samoa. Over half the population is under the age of fifteen years and a strain on land and food resources is beginning to be perceived in some areas of the islands.

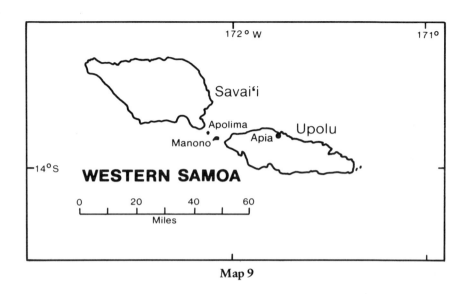

Map 9

In 1976 Apia had a population of approximately 32,000, representing a considerable concentration of people. Although Savai'i is the larger island, it has less than half the population of Upolu and only one thousand more people than the Apia urban area.

The center of the western health service is the National hospital which is situated in Apia. Here all specialist services are concentrated. In 1978 this hospital had 311 beds, with 26 beds allocated to maternity cases.

Babies are usually delivered at the National hospital by qualified nurses who have chosen to concentrate on midwifery. To become nurses the women have trained for three years at the School of Nursing attached to the National hospital. The nurses' training course is adapted to local conditions from the New Zealand nurses' training courses. Supervising midwives have qualifications in midwifery gained from attending postgraduate courses in New Zealand. At the National hospital the midwives do most of the deliveries. But if the health of the mother is in question or if she is either expecting her first child or having her fifth or sixth child, then she is more likely to be delivered by a western-trained doctor.

DEFINITIONS

The World Health Organization (WHO) classifies indigenous midwives such as the *fa'atosaga* in Western Samoa as traditional birth attendants who "mostly have no training at all in midwifery, but are usually well versed in folklore relating to maternal and infant care and are likely to be among the most highly respected members of their communities" (World

Health Organization 1966, 16; and see 1978, 22–27). To WHO "training" means at least secondary school education and some training in scientific medicine.

In 1977 the Department of Health in Western Samoa, following WHO recommendations, introduced a series of one-week courses to provide *fa'atosaga* with some training in western medical procedures relating to midwifery. The courses were held at the district hospitals. The training offered did not fulfill WHO recommendations on education and training, however, so that *fa'atosaga* who took the courses did not attain the WHO-defined status of "midwife."

The introduction of this series of training courses complicates any ethnographic account of midwives and midwifery in Western Samoa. Many Samoan people now make a distinction between a *fa'atosaga* and a "traditional birth attendant" (TBA). *Fa'atosaga* is the term used to refer to midwives who have not attended a Department of Health course, and TBA is the term used to refer to midwives and other women who have attended a Department of Health course. At least one third of the TBAs were not birth attendants before they were selected for the Department of Health courses (Dr. W. Vermuellen, personal communication).

For the purposes of this account the terms *fa'atosaga* and TBA will be used as many Samoan people use them, to differentiate between the two types of indigenous midwives. In Western Samoa the term *fa'atosaga* refers to a position which has been socially differentiated as having specialized status: a *fa'atosaga* is a person who is regarded as a specialist and a professional by herself and her community. Although a distinction is made between *fa'atosaga* and TBA, the positions the terms refer to coincide to a large extent.

INDIGENOUS MIDWIVES

Midwives in Western Samoa are female. The situation sometimes arises where a wife and her husband are both traditional healers who practice together. At a birth the husband assists his wife, who performs the delivery.

Fa'atosaga tend to be elderly and to have had children of their own. Many of them are past menopause. When a woman belongs to a family in which there is a tradition of healing, and she performs her midwifery as part of her healing repertoire, then she may still be of an age to bear children. In contrast, many of the TBAs tend to be women of childbearing age. This contrast results from the way women have been selected for traditional birth attendant courses.

In each village in Western Samoa there is at least one women's committee. The membership of these committees is open to all women but the members are usually women with children, along with a few older high-status women, usually the wives of important village chiefs and orators. The activities of the women's committees include economic projects, activities associated with the well-being of the village, and maternal and child health clinics. Several *fa'atosaga* expressed the view that their midwifery activities prevented them from taking an active role in their women's committee. This was also a reason given for their decision not to go to the traditional birth attendant courses run by the Department of Health. Many of the *fa'atosaga* were approached by district health nurses and invited to go on a TBA course. In villages, even those which have a district hospital or a health clinic, the women's committees are important to the Department of Health. The women who were not *fa'atosaga* and who were selected to go on the traditional birth attendant courses were women who were active members of their local women's committee.

Many *fa'atosaga* are also traditional healers (*fofo* is the term of reference commonly used, *taulasea* is the polite form of address); therefore to distinguish between the ways a person becomes a traditional healer and/or a *fa'atosaga* is difficult. A person may become a traditional healer through supernatural calling, but this is difficult to differentiate from becoming a traditional healer through inheritance, since the supernatural realm is peopled by ancestral spirits. A person may grow up in a family in which there are practicing healers and choose to apprentice herself, or himself, to one of these older relations. Thus inheritance and apprenticeship can be indistinguishable as ways of becoming a traditional healer. Healing skills can also be given by a healer as a *mea'alofa* 'thing of love' to a person who is not kin. This way of becoming a healer can be more clearly identified as an apprenticeship. Usually a *mea'alofa* is given to a person who has been crippled or is chronically ill, that is, a sickly person who has required the frequent attention of a healer.

Regardless of the way in which a person becomes a traditional healer, personal experimentation with herbal remedies and types of massages (*fofo*) is recognized as a characteristic of the practice of healing. Characteristically, too, the ability to heal is recognized as a "gift from God." In most cases the Christian God, rather than an ancestral spirit, is the source to whom this ability is attributed. And the ability to heal, which is God's gift, is the ability to meditate on problems of ill health and to talk sensibly about sickness events with sick people and their families. This Samoan idea of meditation and the ability to speak about sickness is different from the idea of faith healing which westerners equate with a God-given gift for healing and which western observers often project onto nonwestern healing practices.

Not all *fa'atosaga* are traditional healers. The *fa'atosaga* who is not a healer usually identifies her mother as the person from whom she learned her skills and beliefs associated with midwifery. As yet there is no record of a *fa'atosaga* giving her midwifery skills to a person who is not kin, as a *mea'alofa*. However, the traditional birth attendant course is probably acceptable to Samoan people as a way of becoming a midwife because of the tradition that a person can become a traditional healer by virtue of a *mea'alofa* from another healer. This idea is consistent with Samoan villagers' views of the status of traditional healers and western-trained health professionals. Western health professionals are seen as having a similar status to that of traditional healers. They are not accorded the very high status which they enjoy in western societies.

STATUS

The midwife usually occupies a respected position, although some variation in status exists in different villages, depending on whether she is a *fa'atosaga* or a TBA. In one village the *fa'atosaga* was the elderly widowed wife of a man who had held a high-ranking chiefly title. In the same village the TBA, who had become a midwife by attending the Department of Health course, was one of the current holders of the same high chiefly title. The younger woman was the only one who sat in the *fono* 'council of chiefs' on a regular basis. She was also very active in her women's committee. Villagers identified both women as the midwives for the village. At times each of them have been faced with two women delivering at the same time, yet each midwife would attend the two women rather than share their caseload. The two midwives were related, albeit distantly, yet they worked quite separately.

There were several villages in which the advent of the traditional birth attendant courses precipitated a change of status for *fa'atosaga*. Some women's committees decided to fine *fa'atosaga* who refused to go on a Department of Health course and who continued to deliver babies. The *fa'atosaga* reacted in various ways. Some of them continued to provide prenatal and postnatal care but stopped delivering babies, while others were supported by their clientele, who paid the women's committee fine as if it were a fee for a specialized service.

The midwife, in the same way as the traditional healer, has an ambiguous social position. This position results from the way in which Samoan people view sickness *(ma'i)*. Samoan people see sickness as an inevitable, unpredictable, and powerful discontinuity in the flow of life, a disruption of social order. Sickness can destroy both individuals and the groups in which they have membership, the ultimate destruction being the death of an individual and/or the dissolution of a group. But sickness can also create. Pregnancy *(ma'itaga, ma'ito)* is thought of as a sickness. One reason the midwife has high status is that she participates in the treatment of sickness as a creative process. Sickness events can result in a reorganization of the group which is advantageous to everyone concerned.

When a midwife delivers a baby for a family to whom she is not related, she usually receives a gift. This gift includes food (a chicken and/or a taro), a new shirt and skirt, money and/or finemats. The fact that this gift is openly given and received distinguishes midwifery from traditional healing, and *fa'atosaga* and TBAs from traditional healers. Traditional healers believe that if they accept payment for healing a sick person, then, because their healing is a gift from God, they will lose it. In fact, what happens is that members of the sick person's family will leave gifts of food in the back of the house without telling the healer, or give the healer a *pasese* 'money for bus fare'. The healer expresses concern about such gifts but feels that since the gift is a *mea'alofa,* to return or refuse it would be extremely insulting to the giver. On one occasion a healer avoided insulting the patient's family, who gave him money openly, by immediately redistributing it among the people who were with him. He kept nothing for himself. Usually care is taken that such gifts to traditional healers are not openly given or received.

ANTENATAL CARE

One of the most significant differences between TBAs and *fa'atosaga* is in the antenatal care each offers the pregnant woman. For some TBAs, predominantly the ones who were not *fa'atosaga* before attending the Department of Health courses, antenatal care amounts to referring the pregnant woman to the local district hospital for iron tablets. Shortly before the woman is due to deliver, the TBA may massage the woman to ascertain the position of the baby. At this time, if the TBA thinks the delivery may not be straightforward she will refer the woman to the local district hospital. One TBA mentioned a woman whom she had referred to the district hospital but who had ignored her advice. The woman delivered twins with difficulty and one twin died. The TBA thought that she had discharged her responsibility by referring the woman to the hospital. Her attitude toward the woman was not one of sympathy for the loss of the baby, but anger at the stupidity of the woman for not following her advice.

The antenatal care offered by a *fa'atosaga* extends from the time when a woman seeks confirmation of her pregnancy. The *fa'atosaga* identifies pregnancy by gentle abdominal massage. Using massage an experienced *fa'atosaga* can feel the slightest change in the mass of the uterus—this increased mass she identifies as the placenta.

During a woman's months of pregnancy the *fa'atosaga* will massage her abdomen and lower back on many occasions. The massage is intended to relieve any discomfort, to determine the position of the foetus, and to change it if necessary. Clark warns against "the danger of abruptio placentae" (1978, 165) but the antenatal massage I observed was always very gentle, and the *fa'atosaga* constantly asked the woman whether she felt any pain.

As Neich and Neich have noted (1974, 462), a woman's pregnant condition will elicit many comments and statements about pregnancy. The two comments I heard most frequently were that a pregnant woman should never be alone, and that to go out at night is dangerous for a pregnant woman. Neich and Neich's review of the literature shows that, with reference to the statement that a pregnant woman should never be alone,

> Kramer records the prohibition of eating alone, adding that its purpose is to prevent the pregnant woman from eating prohibited food. Mead notes a general prohibition on the pregnant woman to do anything in secret or alone. She suggests that since anything done alone is necessarily shameful or disgraceful, food eaten in private is presumed to be stolen. (Neich and Neich 1974, 462)

And with reference to the statement that to go out at night is dangerous for a pregnant woman,

> a pregnant woman should never be alone in the dark. Otherwise a family *aitu* or other *aitu* 'ghost, spirit' may affect the unborn child. Legends tell of women giving birth to lizards, geckos and other animals as a result of an *aitu* getting near the pregnant woman. A handicap or deformity in a baby could have been caused by an *aitu*. It was said of a still-born deformed baby that the mother must have been out in the night alone, thereby allowing an *aitu* to strangle the baby in the womb. Some informants' statements imply that *aitu* are believed to be active in New Zealand. Goodman says that named *aitu* associated with a particular place are not generally believed to be active in the continental United States, but Samoans there refrain from committing offences against *aitu* said to be spirits of deceased relatives. These latter would presumably also be the *aitu* referred to in New Zealand. The danger of *aitu* to a lone pregnant woman was not mentioned by Mead or Kramer as a reason for keeping the company of others. (Neich and Neich 1974, 462)

The danger of *aitu* 'spirits' to a lone pregnant woman, particularly at night, was the only reason given to me for keeping the company of others. The theme of the conversations in which this statement was made was healing practices and this may have influenced the emphasis placed on the danger of *aitu*. The statement is consistent with the Samoan idea that pregnancy is a sickness. The sick are constantly attended and Samoan people believe that any sickness experience is potentially spirit sickness *(ma'i aitu)*. Every effort is made to prevent the potentiality from becoming a reality; therefore pregnant women should have constant company.

One *fa'atosaga* described, and was observed practicing, a method of contraception. This involved a massage technique which, she said, results in the fallopian tubes being placed so that the ova never find their way to the uterus. This same midwife, massaging a woman, located her IUD and expressed concern verging on horror when told the function of the device. Subsequently she recommended that the woman remove her IUD and return for the contraceptive treatment described here.

The contraceptive method this *fa'atosaga* described is the reverse of one which she and many others use to help infertile women conceive. The treatment begins as soon as the women's next menstrual period finishes. The treatment, given twice a day, involves massaging the fallopian tube into a position which is optimum for receiving the ovum. In addition the *fa'atosaga* counsels the woman's husband, directly if he is present or else through his wife, to have intercourse at a particular time during the month. The reason given for this advice is that intercourse displaces the fallopian tubes to their old position. *Fa'atosaga* do not claim inevitable success for this procedure, but they think they have some. In one village four women with whom I spoke claimed to have become pregnant during the month in which they underwent this treatment.

DELIVERY

In Western Samoa from 1968 to 1978, there was a tendency for more and more women to deliver their babies at the National hospital or at one of the district hospitals. The reversal of this trend since 1978 probably resulted from the recognition on the part of western-trained doctors that their medical facilities could not cope with the demand placed upon them as more and more women came to deliver their babies in the hospital.

In Western Samoa birth is a family affair. There is no seclusion and relatives may attend. A woman expecting her first child is encouraged to return to her mother's home, if this is not her usual place of residence, for the birth of her baby. Subsequent children will be born at the place where she usually resides. While in most villages TBAs and *fa'atosaga* deliver babies in the homes of the women, in some villages TBAs deliver babies in the meeting house of the women's committee.

This account of a delivery was given by a fa'atosaga:

> The first thing I do when a woman comes to me is massage her to make sure the head has turned from an upright position to a downward one. The time when the mother starts to feel the contractions differs for different women.

Some women have mild contractions two weeks before the baby is born. For other women the contractions do not start until a few hours before the baby is delivered. When the woman is in real pain I put in my hand and feel the baby's head. Then I draw down the bag *(lago)* and pinch it to break it.

If the feet come down first I massage the woman's abdomen at the sides to soften the muscles and lessen the contractions. [The *fa'atosaga* demonstrated her massage technique on herself. The first step is gentle massage with hands spread open, which has the effect of vibrating the surface muscles into some degree of numbness. The second step is to stroke the contracted muscles firmly. Once the contractions are lessened the *fa'atosaga* goes back to the baby.] Gently I push the feet back inside and turn the baby with my hand, working on the woman's abdomen. When the baby is ready to come I tell the mother to hold a contraction and the baby slides out. [She showed how the head would be guided by her hand.]

The delivery procedures vary from one *fa'atosaga* or TBA to another. The *fa'atosaga* whose account is given above practices midwifery as part of her repertoire of traditional healing practices. The position in which she delivers a woman varies from woman to woman and with the circumstances relating to the delivery. The woman may deliver lying down or in a sitting position with a pile of pillows behind her back. In each case the *fa'atosaga* sits between the woman's bent legs. Both these positions were described by other *fa'atosaga* and TBAs. One *fa'atosaga*, who was not a traditional healer but who was a *fa'atosaga* before she went on the TBA course, said that if the mother and/or baby becomes tired, then she helps the mother get more out of her contractions by putting the mother's legs over her (the midwife's) shoulders.

Variation also exists in the way *fa'atosaga* and TBAs handle the dilation of the cervix, deal with the amniotic sac, and respond to breech presentations. Most indigenous midwives seem to let the cervix dilate at its own pace; however, one TBA described massaging the cervix to make it bigger if it was tight. Not all midwives break the amniotic sac, but many use their fingers and pinch it to break it. One TBA had a WHO midwifery kit, and she used tweezers to break the membrane. When faced with a breech presentation some midwives followed the procedure described in the account above; others deliver the baby in the breech position. The TBA with the WHO midwifery kit said of breech deliveries, "I thank God for helping me to stay calm. I never panic. If one foot comes down, then I push it back again; if two feet come, I deliver the baby in that position." The midwives' accounts of deliveries indicate that episiotomy is not a part of regular delivery procedure. Nor could I elicit any descriptions of tearing, or possible healing procedures associated with it, such as suturing.

THE PLACENTA AND THE UMBILICAL CORD

Several *fa'atosaga* told stories of women who gave birth attended by their sisters without a *fa'atosaga* present. In each case the delivery was complicated because the expulsion of the placenta *(fanua)* was delayed. The sisters tried to pull the placenta out, but neither their strength nor that of the woman's husband would dislodge it. The family then called in the *fa'atosaga,* who removed the placenta with ease. If the placenta does not respond to gentle massage, then deep, vigorous massage usually dislodges it. This kind of story indicates an awareness among *fa'atosaga* of the potential harm that can be done to the placenta and the uterus by using undisciplined strength or vigorous massage.

Although Cominsky notes "that the placenta is usually expelled without manual assistance" (1976, 240), my experience in Western Samoa suggests that the expulsion of the placenta is usually manually assisted. The *fa'atosaga* whose account of a delivery and breech delivery appears above said:

> I massage the birth passage and the womb in from all sides very, very softly. Then I massage the abdomen using a circular movement. The reason for this is to get the *to'ala* 'life of the abdomen' back into the right place. When I have finished massaging the woman I put two fingers into the womb and pinch the placenta. Once I have hold of it I tell the woman to hold a contraction. While she is holding I pull very gently.

One TBA said:

> When the baby has been born the mother is left for about fifteen minutes. When the mother has pain again I press down and the placenta comes.

And a *fa'atosaga* who had been on a TBA course said:

> To remove the placenta I gently massage the uterus but I never ask the mother to push and then the placenta comes out very easily.

The point in the delivery process at which the umbilical cord is cut varies; sometimes it is before and sometimes it is after the placenta is expelled. Whether the birth is attended by a *fa'atosaga* or a TBA does not influence the point in the process at which the umbilical cord is cut, or in the ideas and practices associated with the cutting of the cord. After the baby is delivered the "life" *(ola)* of the baby is still in the placenta, so the blood *(toto)* or "life" is massaged down the cord into the navel *(pute)*. When the "life" of the placenta has been massaged into the baby, the midwife holds the cord until it stops beating. When the beating stops, a tie is made and the cord is cut. Cotton thread was the material identified for tying the cord. Usually only one tie is made. A razor blade or sharp knife cleaned in hot water is used to make the cut. The distance from the navel where the cut is made varies from one to three inches.

The placenta is disposed of by the *fa'atosaga* and the TBAs in the same way. Nowadays it is carefully thrown into the sea; Samoan people believe that if anything happens to the placenta, something might happen to the baby. I was told that, in the old days, a hole was dug in the ground, a fire was made in the hole, and the placenta was burned before it was buried. The *fa'atosaga* whose account of delivery is given above disposes of the placenta in a different way, more like the old practice. She wraps the placenta in a cloth, and the husband of the mother, or a boy or girl from her family, buries it in the earth *(fanua)*. The word *fanua* means land, field, and afterbirth (Milner 1978, 58).

TREATMENT OF THE NEWBORN

Various rituals are performed to ensure that the baby is breathing. One *fa'atosaga* bounces the baby four times in her hand. If the baby does not begin to breathe, she wraps the baby in a cloth and dips it in cold water; then she dabs it dry with a clean cloth. Samoan babies are usually bathed right after delivery. Many also have Samoan oil rubbed onto them. One *fa'atosaga* puts two drops of oil on the end of the cord. Once bathed, babies are wrapped in a clean cloth and a blanket and laid down to sleep.

Samoan babies are fed on demand. They are fed immediately when they cry. What they are fed varies from one midwife to another. Some recommend breast feeding from birth. Others do not recommend immediate breast feeding; instead they practice a feeding regime in which the baby is first fed on boiled water or coconut milk, for from twelve to five days.

With reference to this feeding pattern Meleiseā (1979, 266–67) discusses the Reverend George Turner's record. She says:

> Turner's opinion that infanticide was not practiced depends on how one interprets the post-natal treatment of newborn infants. He observed that for the first three days after delivery, infants were fed on chewed and strained coconut. On the third day, a "woman of the sacred craft" tested the mother's milk by heating it in a coconut cup two or three times a day for several days. Only when the milk did not "coagulate" was the mother considered ready to begin breast feeding.

Turner (1861, 176) suggested that

only the most robust infants would have survived this type of artificial feeding prolonged over several days, and . . . as a consequence of the custom, the infant mortality rate was high.

That Samoan people were well aware of the consequences of deprivation of breast milk is suggested by the following passage:

Occasionally the father or some member of the family through whom it was supposed that the god of the family spoke, expressly ordered that the [newborn] child have nothing but the breast for an indefinite time. This was a mark of respect to the god and called his "banana." In those cases the child grew amazingly and was soon literally as plump as a banana.

Meleiseā (1979, 266–67) comments:

This form of passive infanticide combined with the absence of modern medical treatment, and the less stable traditional marriage patterns and the traditional prohibition of sexual intercourse between husband and wife during lactation, resulted in a lower birth rate, a smaller number of surviving children born to each woman, and family sizes which rarely exceed four children.

Given Turner's observations and Meleiseā's comments, it is clear that variations in the treatment of the newborn cannot be used as criteria for differentiating *fa'atosaga* and TBAs.

POSTNATAL TREATMENT OF THE MOTHER

Abdominal massage is a central part of the postnatal treatment of the *failele,* the woman who has recently given birth. One *fa'atosaga* said, "I put one hand inside the birth canal and one on the outside and massage the womb *(to'ala fanau)* together." This *fa'atosaga* had already massaged the *to'ala* or "life of the abdomen" into place prior to the expulsion of the placenta.

After the *to'ala* and uterus have been massaged into position, most *failele* are given a bath. Sometimes *failele* are given a bowl of steaming hot water, which they position so that the steam will rise into and cleanse the birth canal.

Then, as in many other cultures (Cominsky 1976, 242), an abdominal binding *(fusi)* is tied around the *failele*'s abdomen. Usually this binding remains in place for about one month. The binding is intended to hold the *to'ala* and uterus in position. If the *failele* is not bound, Samoan women say that the *to'ala* and/or uterus will "fall down," causing lower back pain and pain in the legs on walking.

Once this postnatal treatment is complete the *failele* is given *vaisalo,* which is sago cooked in coconut cream and flavored with lemon leaves.

The convalescent period varies. After the birth of the first child a *failele* is expected to rest for one month; after delivering subsequent babies the *failele* is expected to rest until the newborn baby's cord falls off.

Ma'i o le failelegau is a sickness to which *failele* can be susceptible. Heath says *failelegau* "usually refers to puerperal fever but can refer to any postnatal complication" (1973, 32). *Failelegau* occurs when women work too soon after they have had a baby. They become sick because they have not had enough time to recover properly. To treat this condition an herbal concoction is prepared for the woman to drink.

One *fa'atosaga* described a rare condition she called *tau* which is associated with *failelegau*. She said the stomach becomes as swollen as if the woman were pregnant. To treat this condition, the healer would insert two of her fingers into the *failele's* vagina and manually dilate the cervix. Usually this results in the flow of an unpleasant discharge associated with bleeding. When the flow ends, the healer uses her heel to press down gently into the woman's vagina. In addition to these procedures an herbal douche is prepared from the fleshy inner bark of the *pu'a* tree *(hernandia peltata Meissn.)* (Parham 1972, 103). The treatment of *failelegau* is not the prerogative of the *fa'atosaga* and TBAs, however, and other healers can be involved.

Apart from the payment given to a midwife who is unrelated to the family, no obvious rituals mark the end of the midwife's duties.

CONCLUSION

The TBA courses have added a dimension to the ethnography of midwifery in Western Samoa. The main difference between the TBAs and the *fa'atosaga*, who have not been to a TBA course, is in the practice of antenatal care. The TBAs see the women less often in the antenatal period than do the *fa'atosaga*. The TBA may refer women to the hospital for antenatal care and in those cases where there is a possibility of a complicated delivery. Whether the TBA courses have contributed to any improvements in the birthing process is difficult to decide. The *fa'atosaga* who went on the courses now tend to rely on the district hospitals more than they did before and as a consequence tend to be less confident in their own judgments and practices. In some cases the midwives' tendency to refer women to the hospital rather than treat them themselves interferes with the development of rapport. How this change influences the birthing process has not yet been systematically documented. Apart from antenatal care, no other midwifery practices, beliefs, and attitudes can be used to differentiate TBAs from *fa'atosaga*.

This study of midwifery was carried out in conjunction with more general research into traditional Samoan healing practices. Rather than attempt an exhaustive statement on midwifery in Western Samoa, I have gathered together some of the written sources to elaborate the results of my own fieldwork. More research is needed to understand more fully traditional midwifery in Western Samoa and to appreciate the implications and possibilities of the link that has been created between traditional midwifery and western medical services as a result of the TBA courses.

NOTE

I wish to express my deepest appreciation to the Samoan people who have assisted me in this study. I wish to thank the Government of Western Samoa for permission to carry out this research. My thanks to the Medical Research Council of New Zealand, who funded the fieldwork in Western Samoa, and to Gillian Linney and Jennifer Wood, who typed this manuscript. I acknowledge the Director-General of Health in New Zealand for permission to publish this paper.

11

Notes on Maori Sickness Knowledge and Healing Practices

Claire D. F. Parsons

There are two main views regarding the original medical practices of the Maori people of New Zealand. Some Maoris assert that herbal remedies have always been a major part of Maori healing practices. Others, academics such as Best (1905) and Metge (1978), argue that while some herbal remedies may have been known, Maori sickness explanation limited the exploration of such knowledge.

The Maori people have always had their own healers, known as *tohunga*,[1] who were believed to possess the supernatural power and knowledge to invoke or cure illness. Maori theories of sickness were related to the supernatural world. However, around the turn of the century the Maori population was devastated by epidemics, and to the western medical profession the *tohunga* appeared to be a hindrance to the health of the Maori people (Buck 1966). It was this conflict between differing modes of healing that lead the officer for Maori health, Maui Pomare, to encourage the passing of the Tohunga Suppression Act in 1907, which was not repealed until 1963 (Metge 1978, 94). Though the act was not strictly enforced, the role of the *tohunga* diminished with the inevitable increase of western influence in New Zealand life. Today *tohunga* still exist as healers, often as faith healers using prayer and chant as the major healing skills. They may live in urban centers as well as in country districts. The *tohunga* are highly respected members of any Maori community because of their skills in faith healing, counseling, and Maori medicine.

It is not known how many *tohunga* there are throughout New Zealand. But Maoris other than *tohunga* also practice the art of healing, sometimes using medicinal plants as part of their healing repertoire. Hence, whatever the truth about the history and the extent of herbal

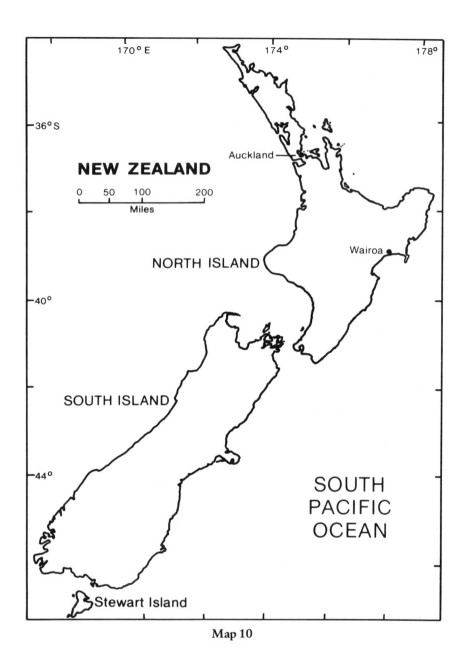

Map 10

remedies being used, they do exist today. Indeed, the interest in locating and documenting such plants is increasing.[2]

Recording the cultural practices of the Maori people is at present a politically sensitive task.[3] With the increase in political consciousness among Maori youth in particular, any European (Pakeha) attempting to document the lifestyle of the urban Maori may meet with considerable resistance. This attitude is not so marked in rural areas where getting to know the people brings amiable discourse and an open exchange of knowledge. The urban resistance is the understandable and inevitable result of the dynamics of social change.

Through this chapter I hope to promote a general awareness of the existence of Maori healing practices and medicines in both rural and urban areas of New Zealand. The chapter is offered as a preliminary discussion rather than a definitive statement. In time, Maori people will make known their own interpretations of their healing practices.

HEALING BELIEFS AND PRACTICES IN A RURAL MAORI COMMUNITY

Wairoa is a rural community on the east coast of New Zealand's North Island.[4] Out of a population of approximately 12,000 (1976 census, Wairoa), 4,607 inhabitants were registered as Maori. While local opinion suggested the ratio of Maori to European was then 50:50, it was understood that a higher number of Maori babies was being born in Wairoa than of any other ethnic group. It is among this steadily increasing Maori population that I sought to understand the knowledge and practices associated with the phenomenon of sickness.

In order to avoid the complexities of the term "perceived morbidity,"[5] the meanings of "health" will be discussed in relation to Maori and European everyday life perspectives. Discussions on health with a group of European New Zealanders will raise questions of diet and exercise and perhaps environmental factors such as fresh air and sunshine. This way of talking about health as a physical dimension of human existence reflects a western perspective. Maori people, however, do not traditionally take this physicalist view. Most Maoris still perceive health (the Maori term *ora* implies spiritual, mental, and physical well-being) in terms of harmonious living—being "at one with" nature, self, and others, although there is much variation in individual philosophies.

Even today the Maori places less emphasis on his or her physical well-being than does the Pakeha. One elder Kahungunu, who had conspicuous shortness of breath and general cyanosis, told me that he had never suffered poor health in his life. He took *karamu* (see Maori Medicines) occasionally but otherwise reported that he had not been sick. This was characteristic of several self-assessments among the adult members of the Ngāti Kahungunu. The general philosophy expresses the feeling that as long as a person is with his (or her) own people and all is well with them, then happiness is assured. Health is thus a way of living. Traditionally, illness was not explained by any disease model but rather as a result of "wrong" living or interference from the spirit world. Such traditional beliefs and perceptions are reflected in the health process and practices of this Maori tribe today. No matter how obese or how many aches and pains experienced, "as long as I can still eat and get about, I am well." Nevertheless, in everyday life illnesses do occur and Kahungunu people widely practice self-medication to alleviate certain discomforts. They are reluctant to consult a doctor and preference is given to natural Maori herbal-botanical decoctions.

The Kahungunu philosophy of death, like their philosophy of life, is at variance with that of the Pakeha. Having highly ritualized the process of death and dying, and having developed strong family and tribal support networks, they are not generally afraid to die as long as, when the time comes, the individual is able to return "home" (meaning the tribal home). "I am happy if I am with my people. I belong somewhere [identity], have my family around me, have enough money to buy food, drink and clothing and know everyone is okay and that I can die at 'home.' I am not worried about anything else. What more is there?"

Of the Maori people interviewed none could name anyone who had ever "suffered from nerves," or been diagnosed by a western doctor as having any form of mental illness. Neither did anyone report knowing anyone in their own tribe who was lonely. One Kahungunu elder said he understood the only cause of mental illness was inherited mental deficiency, although most recognize *mate Maori* 'Maori sickness' (described below). Others know that some people cannot cope with stresses of life but feel that these are the people "trying to live like Pakehas." Thus, when things go wrong the individual turns to family and friends and often to the minister of religion who is sometimes regarded as having *tohunga* status.

As with other cultural groups, divorce and crime are increasing social phenomena among the younger population, and senior members of the Kahungunu point to increasing urbanization (rural-urban drift) and the breakdown of the extended family arrangement as major causes. One person expressed the problem this way: "Young people do not know how to cope with town. They are not prepared for the Pakeha way of life."

There are many sociocultural factors that influence the decision making of Maori people when they perceive themselves to be sick (Parsons 1978). However, I shall confine the discussion here to sickness (more particularly *mākutu),* hospital procedure, the western doctor, alternative healing practices, and Maori medicines.

Sickness, the Supernatural, and Mākutu

Sicknesses are thought to have several causes: accidental (injuries due to accidents); natural (e.g. measles, chicken pox, heart attacks); and supernatural (psychological disturbances often thought to be caused by supernatural forces, possibly as a result of a disturbance in family relationships or a disturbance of spirits of the deceased). Sicknesses involving the supernatural are sometimes referred to as *mate Maori* 'Maori sickness'. In addition, it is sometimes believed that any accident or illness may on occasion be indirectly caused by the supernatural, particularly those which are persistent or not readily diagnosed, and they are also known as *mate Maori.*

Mate Maori is bound up with the traditional belief that illness resulted from "wrong living," especially the breaking of *tapu.* According to tradition, mental anxiety resulting from guilt caused psychosomatic illness, sometimes resulting in death. Ill-luck *(aituaa)* arose not from direct infringement of *tapu* but from a disturbance in the relationships between humans and natural forces. Thus illness and misfortune were associated primarily with the supernatural. Buck (1966) and Metge (1978) present the main causes of Maori sickness as *hara* 'wrong doing', especially breach of *tapu,* and *mākutu,* including what they refer to as "sorcery" (cf. Parsons 1984).

The most conspicuous form of illness caused by intervention of the supernatural was *mākutu,* which still exists today. The supernatural influences of *mākutu* were normally associated with evil. The Kahungunu people sometimes still suspect *mākutu* as the cause of sickness. While many do not directly believe in such forces today, and none said they believed in sorcery, most are still careful not to mock or deliberately transgress situations where there has been the suggestion of an association with *mākutu.* The majority of the Kahungunu still experience what is referred to as "eerie" sensations in certain contexts and know not to ignore such occurrences. As one woman described it, "I don't laugh at it, or ignore it. I respect it. My mother always told us that if ever we get frightened of anything, just stop and say a prayer." This statement is indicative of most attitudes. Another woman, a nursing sister at the local hospital, speaking of her mother's death, described the following incident:

> My mother had been admitted to hospital but as she was told she was dying she was taken home to die. A friend told her she had *mākutu* on her. I brought some arum lilies into the house and was told this was bad luck and something would happen. My mother began to believe there was *mākutu* on her. I growled at her and told her not to be so stupid. A few days later my mother went unconscious. I made my father promise no one was to talk of *mākutu.*

> My father used to sleep with my mother on the couch but one night he went to his own bed to sleep and I was left alone to look after her. That night I had a dream. Two men had black coats on, on a sunny day. I turned around and the two men were standing there. It must have been a dream but I told no one that my mother only had two days to live. She died two days later.

The same woman reported a similar incident, which had occurred only a few days before the interview, involving two people who had come across a disturbed grave while hunting. Instead of burying the exposed bones, one boy picked them up and threw them into the river. His sister told him he would pay for his "wrong." The following week the boy suffered a severe asthmatic attack.

Another recent incident involved a nurse whose boyfriend had died. She had become somewhat irrational and ill. The Maori hospital staff suspected *mākutu* might be involved and that she was "not really ill." The minister of religion was asked to come and say some prayers, which he did. The girl recovered. In this case *mākutu* could be seen as an indication of personal distress.[6]

Spirits are not always seen as malicious, as shown by this account given by another nursing sister.

> One time when I was on night duty, a nursing sister lost a baby [the baby died in the ward while she was on duty] and asked me to accompany her to the morgue. When we got there the trays were full. I pushed one back and put the baby in. When I went back to the wards everything looked okay, but when walking between wards it was like a person was trying to play hide-and-seek with me. I wasn't afraid but about 7.30 A.M. I was coming out of the surgical ward and I met my cousin and her husband and asked what they were doing there. They said they had come to see their child. I said I did not know the child had been admitted or that she had died. I knew then it had been the little girl's spirit playing behind me.

Hospitals and Hospital Procedure

All cultural groups have shared beliefs and superstitions. In European hospitals in New Zealand there are beliefs and superstitions associated with hospitalization, for example that there must be no ward or room number 13, that red and white flowers must not be put together as a bouquet because they signify death, that live patients should be pushed on a trolly head-first and deceased patients feet-first, that prayers should be said at the official opening of a hospital, hospital wing or ward, and so on.

The Ngāti Kahungunu have their own beliefs, which contribute to their reluctance to enter hospitals. Hospitals are managed by Pakehas and most Pakehas are ignorant of Maori values. For example, in hospitals (1) people are admitted to beds where others have died and yet the beds and rooms have not been spiritually cleansed; (2) visiting hours restrict the natural sociability and concern of friends and family, as do the hospital rules allowing only two visitors at the patient's bedside; (3) food is often limited and unpalatable to the cultural tastes of the Maori patient and the preparation of hospital food is often suspect in relation to customary food preparation; (4) the likelihood of having a tray of cooked food passed over one's head (which is *tapu,* thus making it *noa*) adds to the wariness and distress of the Maori patient, especially the elderly patient; (5) confinement to bed preventing the Maori patient from excreting away from the sleeping place is distressing because it violates a *tapu;* (6) all hospital linens are laundered together, a procedure that disregards the Maori distinction between linens used in food preparation and those associated with the body.

Even the hospital's construction can be a cause of concern to Maori people. A number of accounts in Maori legend describe the journey of the *wairua* 'spirit' after it leaves the body, usually said to happen three to five days after death. The Kahungunu believe that departing spirits of the dead move northward to Cape Reinga where they pass down the roots of a tree located on a cliff and enter the underworld. No account tells whether the spirit travels onward to the Maori ancestral home of Hawaiiki or Tawhiti. But in rural communities where traditional practice and beliefs are still strong, the main entrance to buildings, especially hospitals, should, if possible, face north. This prevents spirits traveling north from entering the dwellings. The placement of entrances to the south in hospitals has at times caused concern to Maori people.

Body disfigurement or dismemberment is another cause of distress to the Maori patient, but this is not for cosmetic reasons. Because the Kahungunu believe that in the afterlife one will take the form that one had in the earthly life, the loss of limbs is of great significance. To incinerate dismembered limbs or parts, a conventional hospital practice following surgery or an accident, is to transgress Maori custom. Hence the entrance at Wairoa Hospital, the local hospital for the Kahungunu people, has become the waiting place for relatives to receive amputated limbs to take to the "home" cemetery for appropriate burial. In rural areas today a mother may still request the amputated stump of the umbilical cord, which adjoins the newborn infant to the placenta. Custom decrees the placing of the umbilical cord in a container, usually a bottle, which would be taken to an appropriate repository, often the family cemetery.

Also of concern to Maori patients is their longstanding belief that one is likely to die when admitted to a hospital. This belief is reinforced by the increased chance of death due to the serious condition of the patient as a result of delay. In addition, the belief that it is desirable to be with one's people when dying adds to the reluctance to go to the hospital. Because of such beliefs the Kahungunu people will in many instances attempt self-medication, including home remedies, or simply ignore the condition rather than seek the assistance of the health professional.

Finally, individual hospital policy can have a deterring effect on health service utilization, as did the peculiar system of hospital referral for admission in Wairoa in 1978. In addition to the usual bureaucratic procedures surrounding hospital admission, medical policy insisted that when an ambulance was sent from the hospital (driven by the local taxi driver or even the Matron) to collect a prospective patient, it was necessary that a detour be made to the general practitioner's rooms. The patient had to be taken to his own general practitioner, not another. This detour was for the purposes of assessment and initiation of treatment as well as to gain permission for admission. While such a practice may seem necessary from the doctor's point of view, it also means that the G. P., as the gate-keeper to all health services, is able to collect a fee from this brief encounter. All around, it seems a practice of benefit to the doctor and not the patient.

The Western Doctor

The doctor is actively avoided by Maori people. The residents of Wairoa are expected to register with one practitioner and seek only his advice. But the Maori patient often does not know why he should register with a doctor before he is ill and may not like the manner of the doctor he is assigned to.

Only one of the five practitioners was reported in 1978 to be "good with Maoris," understanding "our ways," and it was suggested that the Kahungunu people sought him out because of this attribute. The general resistance to utilizing doctor services is for the most part due to the lack of understanding of Maori customs on the part of the general practitioner. The increase in use of such services is more often seen among the younger Maori population, especially among mothers with young children.

The use of Practice Nurses operating in the community, exercising fully their diagnostic and therapeutic skills, seems a viable proposition and the Kahungunu people seem most receptive to the idea. Perhaps the Practice Nurses most acceptable to the community would be the Kahungunu nursing staff.

Alternative Healing Practices

Sickness is a phenomenon fundamental to all peoples no matter what their cultural heritage may be. All cultures have institutionalized healing practices, usually with the use of medicines, in an effort to explain and control such phenomena. Therefore many Maori people have not adopted unconditionally western medical practices but have managed an accommodation of both forms of healing art.

Among the Kahungunu there are a certain number of elders, usually women, who still hold the esoteric knowledge of tribal healing practices. The healing skills attributed to these people are acknowledged by those who have had occasion to employ them. Among the Kahungunu there are those who can recount successes (and failures) in healing.

Self-medication is widely practiced and is preferred by most of the Kahungunu to consulting a European doctor. While the younger generation may primarily utilize pharmacological preparations, most adults use conventional Maori medicines.

The minister of religion has a major role as a health advisor. The Kahungunu people do not consider any of their members to be a *tohunga,* although the minister of religion (predominantly Roman Catholic and Church of England) is virtually attributed that status. The minister may frequently be requested to lift *tapu* from material objects (persons, belongings, buildings, land, etc.) that people know, or suspect, to be *tapu.* This is usually achieved through the use of prayer and water.

Prayer and water are commonly used by a Maori who suspects that *tapu* or the supernatural may be involved. In discussion with Maori hospital employees, it was found that both nursing and domiciliary staff frequently say private prayers and wash their hands in situations involving the dying and deceased, or when they experience personal unease or spiritual presences, especially *mākutu*. If such psychological concerns are not relieved they can cause anxiety sufficient to invoke physical illness—and in the past even death. In scientific circles this is known as somatization.

Other possible health resources—chiropractors, color therapists, counselors, crisis centers, women's refuge centers, psychologists, psychiatrists, transcendental or other meditation groups, yoga groups, etc.— were not available in the district. The one physiotherapist in practice was unknown to the people interviewed.

Discussion of what the Kahungunu people do in terms of controlling diet and increasing exercise brought good humored laughter as well as statements about the recognized need to reduce food consumption. In days gone by, the hunting and gathering of food took considerable energy and hence utilized the caloric intake. Today the fish and chip shop and takeout bar is quicker and easier than preparing food at home.

The changing face of the modern family—working wives and the increasing number of single parents living away from the parental home, plus the slowly increasing number of divorced parents—often places the woman in the unenviable position of managing family care and full-time employment, as well as external kinship obligations. While there is social pressure placed on the woman to provide regular home-cooked meals, the takeout meal provides at least some relief from daily chores. Women in these situations appear to experience the poorest health and often chronic fatigue. Some of the women work in excess of a twelve-hour day routinely and others more than an eighteen-hour day where occupational and family commitments are demanding. In instances where there seems to be no way to relieve their problems, such women could be termed "at risk" of deteriorating physical and mental health.

Maori Medicines

I obtained two different kinds of information regarding medicines used by the Maori people of Wairoa. One takes the form of a three-page document put out by The Vegan Welfare and Communication Centre of New Zealand; each of the medications outlined in the document was found to be contained in Christine Macdonald's *Medicines of the Maori* (1973). The other kind of information is based on oral tradition, whereby Maori elders of the Ngāti Kahungunu described to me some of the medicinal preparations currently in use. The parts of the plants selected for use, as well as details of preparation and prescription for specific ills were loosely described as follows.

> God gave man medicines from nature
> HONTI DURI
> *Kahungunu elder*

Blackberry	*dysmenorrhoea*
	Boil the leaves and drink the decoction.
Flax	*hangovers; also used as a purgative*
(harakeke)	Boil the lower part of the leaves and drink half a cup of the juice. It is very bitter but very effective.
Flax roots	*used to expell the placenta (after birth)*
Thistle root	Boil all five ingredients in a tin taking care not to allow the mixture to boil over onto the fire. Boil for three hours. Drink preparation after delivery of the baby.
Plantain weed	
Tutumako	
Dock roots	
Geranium leaves	*poultice for boils, etc.*
	Warm the leaves over a fire, then squeeze out the juice and make a poultice from it.
Karamu	*almost a cure-all (colds, coughs, sore back,*
(Coprosma robusta)	*stomachache, diuresis, etc.)*
	Boil the leaves and drink the decoction.

Kawakawa (*Macropiper excelsum*; Pepper tree)	*boils or cuts; also reported to cure cancer* Boil the leaves and bathe the affected part with the decoction.
Kokomuka	*chafe, rashes, piles, diarrhoea* For chafe, chew the leaves, then apply them to the rash (e.g. on the baby's buttocks). For piles (haemorrhoids), boil the leaves in water, put in a pot, and sit in the water. For diarrhoea, chew three to four leaves and swallow the saliva, then throw the leaves away.
Kowhai (*Sophora tetraptera; Sophora microphylla*)	*broken bones* Scrape the root and then collect the inner bark. Bathe the limbs in the decoction made from boiling the bark.
Manono (*Coprosma australis*)	*eczema, scabies* Scrape the leaves, then apply directly to rash.
Ngaio (*Myoporum laetum*)	*venereal disease* Peel back the bark that is facing the sun. Scrape the inner bark to get enough juice to fill a dessert spoon and drink it [Macdonald 1973 reports this plant as being poisonous]. Repeat daily for two weeks. Do not take any salt while taking the medication as the combination makes it poisonous.
Paewhenua (*Rumex* spp.; Dock)	*eczema* Boil the leaves and apply the preparation to the affected parts.
Pararutiki (Deadly nightshade)	*cuts and lacerations* Boil the plant and apply as a poultice for about ten minutes.
Paratao	*burns* Scrape the inner fleshy root and apply directly to the burn. It has a cooling effect as well as healing properties. Apply twice a day.
Piripiri (*Acaena sanguisorbae*; Bidibid)	*varicosities* Boil the roots and use as a poultice on varicose veins. It relieves discomfort.
Rata (*Metrosideros robusta*)	*venereal disease* Scrape the bark, boil for two to three hours. Drink the juice.

Tanekaha	*as an abortive*
	Boil a small piece of bark cut into strips. Drink the decoction. It is very potent.
Tutu (*Coriaria arborea*)	*abscess*
	Scrape inner bark and boil. Make into a poultice. (It is poisonous to drink causing paralysis and death.)
Violet leaves	*abscess*
	Make a decoction from the leaves and prepare a poultice. Particularly effective for abscess of the breast.

It should be noted that not all of the herbal plants used are native to New Zealand. This demonstrates the experimentation that has taken place in the development of Maori medicines since European contact.

HEALING BELIEFS AND PRACTICES IN SOUTH AUCKLAND

"Street Kids" and Teenage Pregnancy in Urban South Auckland

This urban study is based on my research in 1982 drawn from the experiences reported by Maori women working among Maori youth in the suburbs of South Auckland. "Street kids" is their own term for the teenagers who roam the streets day or night.[7] Many are actually under the age of fourteen and some even under eleven years of age. Some identify more readily with their peers than with their families, from whom they may be estranged. They frequently report themselves the victims of beatings and incest. These teenagers, for a number of reasons, experience disruption in each dimension of their "health" *(ora)*. That is, they experience spiritual, psychosocial, and physical deprivation.

These young people live under houses, in garages, under schools, in cars, or other dubious accommodation. Not surprisingly, such street kids are largely from the lowest socioeconomic and educational level in New Zealand, the majority of Maori descent. Some of the so-called street kids are not permanently on the street but do run away from home on occasion. Both alcohol and drugs—mostly "pinkies" (barbiturates)—are taken. The children sleep in groups and maintain an intense loyalty to each other as group members.

Many of the teenage girls experience the added problem of pregnancy in their early teens. Home remedies for abortion are frequently attempted. Just as frequently, the child is carried to full term. Occasionally a young, pregnant Maori girl will turn up at an antenatal clinic—sometimes having been coerced by family and friends to attend—and confides her experiences to one of the Maori nursing sisters. From such confidences comes the occasional report that a grandmother, or aunty, has prepared a "medicine" to prevent pregnancy. If the girl becomes pregnant in spite of the medicine, the rationale is sometimes given that insufficient was taken or that it was not taken as prescribed. Reportedly, approximately twenty (predominantly Maori) street girls have turned up at a particular antenatal clinic in Auckland in the four to six months during the winter of 1982. According to their comments, other girls have effectively aborted their babies.

After a girl delivers her baby she may decide not to go back to the street, returning home or to a woman who may have taken her in and cared for her in late pregnancy. Girls who have completely lost contact with their families have no access to contraceptive, abortive, or other herbal remedies of their Maori kinfolk. Others do maintain some family contact, often with a grandmother who has a special rapport with her *mokopuna* 'grandchild'. It is often she who provides, or has access to, medicinal preparations. The mother, still of childbearing age herself, is generally either unfamiliar with the preparations or not in her daughter's confidence.

One fourteen-year-old girl, late in pregnancy, arrived at the antenatal clinic. She confided that her grandmother had boiled a brew from the bark of a tree (she thought it was the *kawakawa* tree) and had offered the medicine as a contraceptive. The woman had told her two granddaughters to drink the medicine after "having sex." The older of the two girls had managed to avoid pregnancy for several years, however, the younger did become pregnant. In the young girl's words, "Nana couldn't keep up with the demand!" My informant suggested with amusement that "Nana" must have ring-barked every tree of that kind in Auckland.

A common interest among the girls and their grandmothers seems to be the "feel" and "lie" of the baby, and palpating the girl's abdomen is part of the overall interest in the development of the baby. Some girls say their grandmother can tell the sex of the baby through palpation and such is the trust in the grandmother's experience and knowledge that, reportedly, a girl may be quite disappointed or mystified when she delivers a baby of the opposite (unexpected) sex.

Some of the grandmothers are also reported as being concerned to turn the baby. Using oil and massage the baby may be gently turned to the cephalic, head first, or breech, buttock first, presentation. In some families, and indeed among some tribes, a breech birth is considered preferable, the explanation being that the more "defiant" entry into the world means a stronger character will develop.

Maori medicines for morning sickness were not reported, possibly as a result of the girls' belated arrival at the clinic. However, my informant said that most Maori women expect to be sick when pregnant. This expectation, more prevalent among Maori women than western, possibly reflects their more negative antenatal experience as a minority group.

As research on Maori women's health shows, these young women are more likely to be aggravating their condition by heavily smoking and taking alcohol or drugs.

Although their attendance at antenatal clinics and classes is erratic, the girls manage to arrive at the hospital for the delivery of their child. Because hospital deliveries are most common, Maori medicines for postnatal recovery are unreported. However, three Maori medicines were reported as being frequently used at other times in the reproductive cycle.

1. Roots of flax (*Phormium tenax;* native New Zealand flax) are boiled and the mixture drunk as prescribed. It is said to control the menstrual cycle and is used as an abortive.
2. *Kumarahou (Pomaderris kumeraho)* is possibly the most common ingredient used in South Auckland for Maori medicine. *Kumarahou* is prepared in several ways and given for various conditions. One use described is for the treatment of uterine pains and/or menstrual pains.
3. *Mamaku* fern *(Cyathea medullaris)* is collected and the fern stem split to remove the pith. This pith is made into a poultice for the treatment of breast abscesses. It is believed to cure cancerous lumps, though these are from the western clinical viewpoint more likely to be breast abscesses or congestion in young postnatal girls.

Such preparations are often taken without knowledge of their actual ingredients. This is especially the case with teenage girls.

Other practices by Maori mothers affecting the newborn child, or later child development, are not necessarily confined to the street girl mother. Clubfoot babies, babies born with the foot rotating inward or outward, are sometimes regarded by Maori mothers as more suitably treated by massage and corrective stretching of the foot rather than with the application of plaster of paris boots, the western orthopaedic healing practice. Some mothers will remove the plasters applied at the orthopaedic clinic in favor of their own therapy. Massage is used extensively for any part of the body causing discomfort, for children and adults alike, therapeutically and socially. There is a higher level of physical contact among Maoris than Pakehas, and therefore massage is culturally appropriate.

Another practice considered to be Maori is the burial of the placenta. Unlike the Kahungunu, a mother or father, or a member of the immediate family, may occasionally request the whole placenta or afterbirth. In one reported case, the placenta of the child was taken home from the hospital in a plastic bag and frozen in the freezer until the family was ready to visit the home marae (tribal homeland) to bury it in the cemetery. The practice is believed to strengthen the child's tie to the land. The placenta is part of the person, like an arm or leg, and it is not considered appropriate to simply discard it. I have also heard of this custom among particular Maoris living in the rural areas of the North Island's east coast. In urban areas, the placenta may be buried under a tree rather than taken home (the home marae) to be buried.

The John Waititi Marae (Inc. Soc.) and Maori Healing Practices in South Auckland

This marae in urban Auckland was founded to promote cultural learning for the enhancement of mutual Maori-Pakeha understanding. It supports a variety of cultural programs encouraging the retention of Maori skills, knowledge, and arts, collectively referred to by Maori and Pakeha alike as *maoritanga*.

One of the activities, incidental to the organized programs of the marae, is the practice of Maori medicine. Healers treat physical and mental disorders by various means. Approximately six women in association with the marae are permanently involved in the preparation of medicines: the gathering of plants (leaves, roots, barks) and the formulation of prescriptive ingredients. *Kumarahou* and other leaves are frequently collected and stored at the John Waititi marae. The women treat conditions such as bladder problems, rashes, respiratory complaints, cuts, burns, bruises, breast abscesses, genito-urinary discharges, sprains, and so on.

These women have their own methods of making preparations. *Kumarahou* is possibly the most common ingredient used; *karamu* is another common ingredient of herbal remedies. One such remedy is used to treat bladder trouble. *Karamu* is collected and combined with wild broom. These ingredients are boiled and the liquid is then ingested in several dosages. The mixture reportedly increases the yellowness of urine, but its active ingredients are thought to "clean away" any urinary infection or irritation. *Tutu* leaf is used to "dry up" weeping rashes, and a mixture of *kumarahou* and *kawakawa* as a remedy for "bronchitis." *Kumarahou* is considered by one healer to be sufficient for the treatment of coughs. For "broken bones" (my western interpretation would suggest some disorder like a sprain), *tupakihi* is collected from the bush. It may be combined with eucalyptus gum for its pleasant odor and is then applied externally. A reported remedy for open sores is a preparation made from scraped and boiled *tawhero*. It is said that three applications will cure the problem.

Actual ingredients and methods of preparing medicinal (herbal) remedies are often considered secret. A number of reasons are given for this: from a woman at the marae (1) "People don't want to be thought to be stupid, or thought to have foolish practices"; and (2) There is "a personal mysticism and prestige as a result of knowing the prescriptions"; a young Maori activist states that (3) "Maori people know the remedies are effective and do not need western science to prove it. They are not concerned with Pakeha approval or proof of the effectiveness of Maori medicine"; and (4) "By informing the Pakeha, commercial gain may be made by the Pakeha of such effective preparations." The secret knowledge of Maori medicine is held by certain members of particular families, and people know through their communication networks who to seek for particular cures. What is unknown, even to the Maori people, is the actual number of Maoris preparing and administering Maori medicine either in Auckland or in New Zealand as a whole. Opinions such as "there are a lot in Auckland alone" are impossible to translate into quantifiable terms, but the opinion is nonetheless significant.

Some Maori people assert there to be not only lay healers but also *tohunga* practicing their healing skills in Auckland. Male and female Maori healers may treat a sick person of either sex. The physical disorders may be treated with herbal remedies or massage, psychological disorders by chant, prayer and water, or counseling.

Such informal counseling may be the major aspect of healing in the Waititi marae, though it may be thought of simply as "helping someone who needs help." Counseling may be in the form of discussions or group therapy. Frequently a young Maori is counseled by an elder. Workers involved in the marae treat many "psychological disorders" and such counseling can be understood as a significant dimension to healing skills practiced in the marae.

Throughout New Zealand no charge is made for Maori healing services. A *koha* 'gift' may be given, though not expected, for services rendered. The women at the John Waititi marae freely give their healing services to anyone who requests them. The healers at the marae are not necessarily known as either *tohunga* or as healers. They are simply people, often women, who are known to have particular cures for particular ills.

Other Maori people in the South Auckland community are faith-healers who may combine prayer, chant, and water. Still others practice psychic healing. Psychic healers may advertise that they are healers in that particular craft and there are, reportedly, an increasing number of Maoris who prefer that alternative. Faith healing is attractive, particularly for those of the Ringatū faith. The Ringatū church was founded by Te Kooti in the 1870s among people on the east coast of New Zealand's North Island long after Europeans had arrived. Faith healers and psychic healers have beliefs and practices analogous to the Ringatū. Chanting is combined with the prayers of faith healing to assist and strengthen the sick person. Practices of both western medicine and Maori medicine may be combined with this.

Maoris in general frequently regard water as having a significant ritual cleansing power. The water need not be "blessed" by a minister of religion. It may simply be tap water. The cleansing power is located in the ritual of its application, for example, the washing of hands, the sprinkling of a house or of one's own body, or another's, as a spiritual cleansing following a death. There is some tribal and religious variation in the importance placed on the cleansing power of water. Such expressions of cultural and religious belief are important for the mental health of the people.

An example of psychologically induced illness can be seen in the following account of a Ringatū penny.[8] In 1982 a woman of the Ratana faith[9] was given a Ringatū penny. Not being of the Ringatū faith she was not attentive to the special care required of such articles and that day placed the penny on top of a wardrobe in her home. Three days later her husband was admitted to an Auckland hospital with a heart condition and was found to have an enlarged heart. The woman felt there was a relationship between her husband's illness and her disregard of the Ringatū penny. She decided to take the penny and bury it. Afterward, she noted a marked improvement in her husband's condition and attributed it to her own action. My informant, an East Coast Maori herself, remembered that when children occasionally found a Ringatū penny they would be instructed to throw it out to sea.

In sum, Maori healing practices are both available and in use, not only in the rural areas but also in highly urbanized areas such as Auckland. Both physical healing skills (herbal remedies, massage) and psychological skills (counseling, chants, prayers, psychic and faith healing) are available to the Maori who is experiencing sickness.

Case Studies

The following are three accounts of personal experiences involving sickness, recorded and translated by a Maori university lecturer in 1982, in the Auckland area. Although she did not wish to be identified, she felt her transcripts showed aspects of sickness, healing, and practices of the *tohunga*.

Informant 1. I am sixty-five years old and come from Te Hapua. At the age of seventeen I left Te Hapua to marry and settle in the Hastings area. My tribe is Te Aupouri and in moving away from my place of birth after my parents were killed by the epidemic [influenza] about 1918, I was bereft of much of the cultural and social awareness of my people. In looking back from my last seventeen years I have no recollection of any sort of healing practices in the community. There were no instances of *mākutu* or black magic—the Maori term was little used by the Maori-speaking community which lived in complete isolation while I lived there and well into the period before the Second World War.

This was in direct contrast to the community that I married into. The concept and practice of *mākutu* was very much a part of the life-style of the people. Practitioners were known by the locals and farther afield, depending on their effectiveness in terms of healing cases of *mate Maori* or Maori sickness.

I have witnessed and known of many cases where Maori patients, suffering from complaints that the general medical practitioner could not diagnose and cure, have resorted to consulting the *tohunga*. In general the procedure is one where the *tohunga* is called or consulted. The patient is often attended by several kin who sit about the room or house where the patient is. There is always a concentrated concern for the patient. There are prayers intoned by different members present. The atmosphere is one of tension and apprehension. I often felt in such situations that the patient became psychologically affected by the presence of the assembled kin. The *tohunga* appears to wait or may be timing the playing of his role at this point in the patient's condition.

Different *tohunga* perform their roles in different ways. All appear however to intone Maori chants or Christian prayers endlessly. Some quote texts from the Bible while standing over the patients and in the presence of others. Others chant and pray well away from the patients but in the same room. Others indeed perform this task in an adjacent room.

In some instances if the patient does not respond he or she is taken to another *tohunga* who may be some distance away and believed to have greater powers. In such an event the patient is again accompanied by senior kin. The local expert or *tohunga* remains but continues to concentrate on his ex-patient. A feature of such involvement which always intrigued me was the follow-up by the *tohunga* once the patient recovers or appears to recover. Kin are questioned on all matters concerning the family—whether the patient visited a marae, partook of some food from a stranger, had something in the house that belonged to another person. . . . Through such queries I have known *tohunga*s to enter the patient's home and pick up some insignificant article—a pencil, bead, ribbon etc.—and indicate that the problem lies with it. Often the article leads the *tohunga* to the person who he believes is the source of the patient's illness. The article is often chanted over by the *tohunga,* so removing its connection with the person who owns it. Once it is made ineffective the patient shows signs of recovery. In all instances of *tohunga* performing their roles they invariably go into what appears to be a trance, quite unaware of who or what is around them. At the end of their vigil they are often wet with perspiration and look very calm and rested, as if awakened from a deep sleep.

I have firsthand experience in Maori healing—I suffered from poor circulation in my legs to the extent that I developed ulcers. My legs discolored until they went the color of dried blood. I made an appointment with a *tohunga* in Auckland. I was unable to walk, and moved around for approximately three months on my knees.

On the first day I reported to the *tohunga*, a woman, at 9:00 A.M. Sat and talked with other patients all day. Went home at 4:00 P.M. after meeting the *tohunga* who asked that I return the next day with some crabs in a jar.

On the second day I reported to the *tohunga* with a jar of crabs. Eventually sat with *tohunga*. She read a chapter from the Bible which for me was my past life history. I was amazed to hear a perfect stranger telling me all about my wretched married life. Having completed the reading she then went into a trance, a deep trance. Then she came to and asked for the crabs, and asking how many ulcers there were, since both my legs were bandaged up. I indicated that there were three. On taking the crabs out of the jar she revealed I had got the right number. There were three, one for each ulcer. She allowed the crabs to run over my bandaged legs, then replaced them in the jar and instructed they be returned to the beach where they belonged. I was given two half-gallon jars of concoctions brewed from the broom plant which I had to take daily. Once drunk, I had to collect the leaves of different native trees, shrubs, and boil them in water. This I drank for the next three months. My circulation and blood improved and the ulcers healed. In two months I was walking and did not require my walking sticks.

Informant 2. I am a hyperactive woman of forty years with a family of three boys and two girls. The youngest of the family are attending intermediate school. I have worked in the Department of Maori Affairs for approximately five years. In this time I have had increasing discomfort with my periods. I suffered from anemia. More and more it seemed that by Christmas of each year I was over-tired. I suffered from bad headaches, my periods were very heavy. I did not eat well. I was over-anxious and got very depressed. I consulted my family doctor who recommended that I take a course of iron pills in preparation for a hysterectomy in March of the following year. My condition worsened. By Christmas I went away for a break. While away I was persuaded to visit a local *tohunga* [a woman].

I had grown up in Auckland so I had little awareness of the *tohunga* scene. However I was so poorly, my husband and I made an appointment for me to see the *tohunga*.

On the first day I went to the house of the *tohunga*. After asking a few questions to appreciate my state of health she prayed over me in the Christian manner. She indicated there was no need for me to continue with the iron pills. She did not recommend a hysterectomy. I returned home with instructions to call again the following day.

On the second day I woke up. Was very depressed. My mother and my husband became concerned for me. The *tohunga* was consulted and she advised that I report that morning. I did. The *tohunga* made the point that since her Christian prayers had had no effect, she believed that my condition was Maori based, *mate Maori*. My husband sat while the *tohunga* concentrated on me. She began praying in Maori, then moved to an adjacent room. She washed her hands and still praying she went into a deep trance placing and running her hands over the whole of my head. That part of my head that ached whenever I went cold and chilled. I drifted off into a deep sleep. It was a wonderfully soothing sensation and I had no wish whatever to "come to." When I did it was to realize that my husband, a big, heavyset man, was trembling all over. And to my amazement tears ran down his face. He was completely overcome. We were required to sit and remain with the *tohunga* for the rest of the day.

That next day we traveled back to Auckland. In a matter of a week I was on top of the world, eating and sleeping well. I was much more relaxed than previously. I was no longer anemic and the color came back into my face very quickly. On returning to work my colleagues were amazed at the improvement in my health. All had been concerned prior to Christmas. I had commented to my aunt that I could not accept the fact my illness was Maori based. She in turn reminded me I was working among Maoris who were from other tribes and therefore the possibilities were there. Her thinking was supported by another elder of mine who lunched with me afterward. On learning of my experience with the *tohunga* she offered the comment that she knew about it, and what's more, she knew the person responsible. He was male and was from another tribe and had been psyching me for some time but unknown to me, the victim.

While I was dumbfounded by this revelation, I was at the same time content and satisfied with my lot. I accepted the fact that there were strong, positive forces about me—all was well with the world and I had nothing to worry about.

My condition remained stable until I ran myself into the ground again through overwork.

Informant 3. I am a member of the Ringatū faith. I grew up steeped in *tohunga*ism. My community accepted the *tohunga* and the role that he played. As an elder of the community I was conscious of all occasions when a member within our ranks became ill; or when there was a birth or death. On such occasions the Ringatū protocol came into play. Prayers and incantations were said and chanted. The *tohunga*, or *tohunga*s, would join the kin who came together as one. On such occasions the *tohunga* would at times take the patient to running water and would sprinkle him with it—a cleansing of the patient of negative elements. The running water, the power, is harnessed to remove it.

Another common practice used by us of the Ringatū faith was the use of pennies on patients who have to be admitted to the hospital, a foreign institution. Such patients have to be cleared of ties with the Maori "connection" so that the Pakeha approach is unhindered. Such patients would have pennies placed on his body, the belief being that such foreign matter has the power and ability to destroy the Maori connection. Once completed, the coins were either thrown into the sea or into a cemetery where no one can reach them. The Ringatū adherents traditionally bathe in running water. The use of hot water is unheard of.

CONCLUSION

While Maori herbal medicines have apparently developed since the days of their contact with Europeans, the role of the Maori healer seems to have existed long before their arrival due to the need to explain the phenomenon of sickness. Originally designated as *tohunga,* the healer role has been extended to those not only of traditional *tohunga* status but to those with sufficient expertise to be regarded as healers. The Maori healer today has a repertoire of healing skills still of relevance to the Maori people. From the descriptions given in this article, the Maori healer is considered to offer an effective practice to both the rural and urban Maori, even where western health services are readily available. Some Maoris will use Maori medicine while others will try western medicine as their first option for minor physical ills or those thought to be of a psychological nature. Most Maori people in urban areas will turn to western medicine for treatment of a serious illness. However, in instances where chronic illness develops, a combination of Maori and western medicine may be seen as the most pragmatic course to relieve distress or discomfort.

In order to understand the reasons for the continuance of this alternative to western medicine, it is necessary to understand Maori sickness explanations in far greater depth than I have been able to present here. It is also necessary to understand Maori resistance to the western healer who is unable or unwilling to demonstrate a culturally sensitive approach in his service to the sick.

NOTES

1. The term *tohunga* is most correctly used with a qualifier indicating the specialty of the particular *tohunga: tohunga taa moko* 'tattooing expert', *tohunga taarai waka* 'canoe making expert', and so on. The term is sometimes loosely applied to anyone skilled in a particular craft, but it is usually reserved for those who are believed to have a special spiritual power associated with their knowledge or skills.

2. Recently an attempt was made by a Maori member of Parliament, Dr. Bruce Gregory, to pass legislation to ensure that such a documentation of Maori medicines be undertaken (see *New Zealand Herald,* Friday, 7 May 1982). The bill was not passed, although the attempt is still being pursued.

3. The original Maori author of this chapter, because of unusual circumstances, was unable to contribute to the book. To fill the gap I have salvaged notes collected over the past four years. Deficiencies in details and continuity of research are a result of this situation. What has emerged is chapter which compares notes on contemporary Maori healing practices in a rural-urban setting with those in a highly urban setting.

4. I am grateful for the assistance of Viv Newman and the members of the Ngāti Kahungunu tribe who participated in the study. I am also grateful to members of the John Waititi Marae, Auckland, and to those of the Maori people who graciously assisted me yet wished to remain anonymous. I wish to thank the Medical Research Council of New Zealand, which provided the "seed money" to support my research among the Ngāti Kahungunu people in 1978.

5. See Parsons 1978.

6. Where distress is somatized (giving rise to bodily symptoms), it acts as a "metaphor for personal distress" (Katon, Kleinman, and Rosen 1982, 246). It may be that the majority of instances of reported *mākutu* are indeed a somatization of psychological distress.

7. Today the number of Maori and other Polynesian and European street kids has increased and in some instances it has become a fashionable form of rebellion among the young. Some of the practices here described are specific to the physical and mental remedies available to the Maori street kids; some are available to Maori women in general. Postnatal practices relating to child development (clubfeet, care of the placenta, etc.), while spoken of in relation to the discussion on street girls, are practices familiar to other women in South Auckland.

8. A Ringatū penny is one which has been burnt, symbolic of days of conflict between Maori and Pakeha. Evil powers or spirits causing sickness *(mākutu)* were driven into the penny, a symbol of Pakeha material evils, and through the biblical purification of fire the evils were ritually destroyed. The act leaves a residual effect of *tapu* in the penny. This form of sacrificial offering is still practiced today. Such pennies are believed to contain the supernatural powers associated with all *tapu* objects.

9. The Ratana and the Ringatū faiths are the two predominant Maori religious denominations, though most Maoris belong to the European denominations, and some combine a European and a Maori faith.

References

Argyris, Chris, and Donald A. Schon
    1976   *Theory in Practice: Increasing Professional Efficiency.* San Francisco: Jossey Bass Pub.

Barrau, Jacques
    1961   *Subsistence Agriculture in Polynesia and Micronesia.* Bernice P. Bishop Museum Bulletin no. 223. Honolulu: Bishop Museum Press.

Beaglehole, Ernest, and Pearl Beaglehole
    1938   *Ethnology of Pukapuka.* Bernice P. Bishop Museum Bulletin no. 150. Honolulu: Bishop Museum Press.
    n.d.   *Myths, Stories and Chants from Pukapuka.* Manuscript in Bernice P. Bishop Museum Library, Honolulu.

Beaglehole, John Cawte, ed.
    1962   *The Endeavour Journal of Joseph Banks, 1768–1771.* 2 vols. Sydney: Angus and Robertson.

Beaglehole, Robert et al.
    1980   Death in the South Pacific. *New Zealand Medical Journal* 91 (660): 375–78.

Beckett, Jeremy
    1964   Social Change in Pukapuka. *Journal of the Polynesian Society* 73:411–30.

Bedford, Richard, Barrie MacDonald, and Doug Munro
    1980   Population Estimates For Kiribati and Tuvalu 1850–1900: Review and Speculation. *Journal of the Polynesian Society* 89:199–246.

Best, Elsdon
    1905   Maori Medical Lore. *Journal of the Polynesian Society* 14:1–23.

Biggs, Bruce, and Mary Veremalumu Biggs
    1975   *Na Ciri Kalia: The Oral Traditions of Cikobia-i-ra.* Working paper no. 42. Anthropology Department, University of Auckland.

Brady, Ivan
    1975   Christians, Pagans and Government Men: Culture Change in the Ellice Islands. In *A Reader in Culture Change.* Vol. 2, *Case Studies,* ed. Ivan A. Brady and Barry L. Isaacs, 111–45. Cambridge, Mass.: Schenkman Pub. Co.

Brodie, Walter
    n.d.   The Brodie Papers: Extracts From Journals. Typescript in the Alexander Turnbull Library, Wellington.

Buck, Peter
    1966   *The Coming of the Maori.* Wellington: Whitcombe and Tombs Ltd.

Burrows, Edwin Grant
    1936   *Ethnology of Futuna.* Bernice P. Bishop Museum Bulletin no. 138. Honolulu: Bishop Museum Press.
    1937   *Ethnology of Uvea (Wallis Island).* Bernice P. Bishop Museum Bulletin no. 145. Honolulu: Bishop Museum Press.

Chabouis, L.
    n.d.   *Petite histoire naturelle de la Polynésie français.* Vol. 1, *Botanique;* vol. 2, *Zoologie.* Papeete: La Société Polynésienne d'Édition.

Chalmers, James
    1870   South Seas Letters, August 15, 1870. London Missionary Society Records Relating to the South Seas, 1796–1899.

Chambers, Anne
    1975   *Nanumea Report: A Socio-economic Study of Nanumea Atoll, Tuvalu.* Rural Socio-economic survey of the Gilbert and Ellice Islands. Department of Geography, Victoria University, Wellington [2nd ed. Canberra, Australian National University, Development Studies Centre, 1984].

Chambers, Keith, and Anne Chambers
    1975   Comment: A Note on the Ellice Referendum. *Pacific Viewpoint* 16:221–22.

Clark, Ann
    1978   The American Samoan. In *Culture, Childbearing, Health Professionals,* ed. A. Clark. Philadelphia: F. A. Davis Co.

Collocott, Ernest
    1923   Sickness, Ghosts and Medicine in Tonga. *Journal of the Polynesian Society* 32 (no. 3): 136–42.

Cominsky, Sheila
    1976   Cross-cultural Perspectives on Midwifery. In *Medical Anthropology,* ed. Francis X. Grolig, S. Harold, and B. Italey. The Hague: Mouton Pub.

Department of Health
    1978   *Annual Report of the Department of Health.* Apia: Government of Western Samoa.

Department of Statistics
  1979   *Quarterly Statistical Bulletin.* 2nd quarter, April-June. Apia: Government of Western Samoa.
Dingwall, Robert
  1976   *Aspects of Illness.* London: Martin Robertson and Co. Ltd.
Ellis, William
  1853   *Polynesian Researches During a Residence of Nearly Eight Years in the Society and Sandwich Islands.* 2nd ed. 4 vols. London: Henry G. Bohn.
Fabrega, Horacio
  1972   Concepts of Disease: Logical Features and Social Implications. *Perspectives in Biology and Medicine* (Summer 1972): 583–615.
Firth, Raymond
  1936   *We, The Tikopia.* London: George Allen and Unwin, Ltd.
  1948   Religious Belief and Personal Adjustment. *Journal of the Royal Anthropological Institute* 78:25–43.
  1959   *Social Change in Tikopia.* London: George Allen and Unwin, Ltd.
  1967   *Tikopia Ritual and Belief.* London: George Allen and Unwin, Ltd.
  1970   *Rank and Religion in Tikopia.* London: George Allen and Unwin, Ltd.
Foster, George
  1976   Disease Etiologies in Non-Western Medical Systems. *American Anthropologist* 78:773–82.
Gaillot, Marcel
  1962   La Circoncision à Futuna. *Journal de la Société des Océanistes* 18: 207.
Garfinkel, Harold
  1967   *Studies in Ethnomethodology.* Englewood Cliffs: Prentice Hall.
Gifford, Edward
  1929   *Tongan Society.* Bernice P. Bishop Museum Bulletin no. 61. Honolulu: Bishop Museum Press.
Gilbert and Ellice Islands Colony
  1944–   Annual Reports (Native Government), Nanumea. Gilbert and Ellice
  1967   Islands Colony file 34/10/17, Reports and Returns. Consulted at Western Pacific Archives, Suva, Fiji.
  1950   Ellice District Annual Reports. District Report for 1950. Gilbert and Ellice Islands Colony file 3/1/6, vol. 2. Consulted at Western Pacific Archives, Suva, Fiji.
Gill, William
  1862   South Seas Letters, Sydney, July 16, 1862. London Missionary Society Records Relating to the South Seas, 1796–1899.
  1877   Visit to Outstations, July 3 to August 14, South Seas Journals. London Missionary Society Records Relating to the South Seas, 1796–1899.

1879 Journal of a Voyage in the *John Williams* to the Outstations of the Hervey Group, August 19 to September 1879, South Seas Journals. London Missionary Society Records Relating to the South Seas, 1796–1899.

Gilson, Richard Phillip
1970 *Samoa 1830–1900: The Politics of a Multi-Cultural Community.* Melbourne: Oxford University Press.

Glick, Leonard
1967 Medicine as an Ethnographic Category: The Gimi of the New Guinea Highlands. *Ethnology* 6:31–56.

Gonzalez, Nancie Solien
1966 Health Behaviour in Cross-Cultural Perspective: A Guatemalan Example. *Human Organization* 25:122–25.

Goodman, Richard A.
1971 Some *Aitu* Beliefs of Modern Samoans. *Journal of the Polynesian Society* 80:463–79.

Goupil, Sarah
1926 Médecines tahitiennes. Raau. *Bulletin de la Société d'Études Océaniennes* 2:95–97.

Grézel, Isidore
1878 *Dictionnaire futunien-français avec notes grammaticales.* Paris.

Gudgeon, W.
1909 Resident Commissioner of the Cook Islands, Report for the Year Ending 31st March 1909. Included in the New Zealand Parliamentary Papers A3, Session II, 1909:6.

Hammond, Dorothy
1970 Magic: A Problem in Semantics. *American Anthropologist* 72:1349–56.

Heath, Timothy
1973 The Diagnosis and Treatment of Disease in a Rural Village in Western Samoa. M.A. thesis, University of Auckland.

Hecht, Julia
1976 Double Descent and Cultural Symbolism in Pukapuka, Northern Cook Islands. Ph.D. diss., University of Chicago.
1977 The Culture of Gender in Pukapuka: Male, Female and the Mayakitanga 'Sacred Maid'. *Journal of the Polynesian Society* 87:183–206.
1978 "Let's Go to Pukapuka": The Home Island and Homes Away From Home. Revised paper presented at the 6th Annual Meeting of the Association of Social Anthropology in Oceania, Monterey, California, 1977.
1981 The Cultural Contexts of Siblingship in Pukapuka. In *Siblingship in Oceania: Studies in the Meaning of Kinship,* ed. Mac Marshall. Association for Social Anthropology in Oceania Monographs no. 8. Ann Arbor: University of Michigan Press.

Hocart, A. M.
   1929   *Lau Islands, Fiji.* Bernice P. Bishop Museum Bulletin no. 62. Honolulu: Bishop Museum Press.

Hooper, Antony
   1975   Review Article of Robert Levy's "Tahitians." *Journal of the Polynesian Society* 84:369–78.

Katon, W., A. Kleinman, and G. Rosen.
   1982   Depression and Somatization. *The American Journal of Medicine* 72 (1): 127–35; (2): 241–47.

Keesing, Felix M.
   1934   *Modern Samoa: Its Government and Changing Life.* London: George Allen and Unwin, Ltd.

Kennedy, Donald
   1931   *Field Notes on the Culture of Vaitupu, Ellice Islands.* Memoirs of the Polynesian Society no. 9. New Plymouth, New Zealand: The Polynesian Society.

Kirch, Patrick V.
   1976   *Cultural Adaptation and Ecology in Western Polynesia: An Ethnoarchaeological Study.* Ann Arbor: University Microfilms.

Kleinman, Arthur
   1980   *Patients and Healers in the Context of Culture: An Exploration of the Borderland between Anthropology, Medicine and Psychiatry.* Berkeley: University of California Press.

Kofe, Laumua
   1976   The Tuvalu Church: A Socio-historical Survey of Its Development Towards an Indigenous Church. Bachelor of Divinity thesis, Pacific Theological College, Suva, Fiji.

Kramer, Augustin
   1941   *The Samoan Islands.* Trans. D. and M. de Beer. Apia, Western Samoa: Department of Native Affairs.

Lemaitre, Y.
   1973   *Lexique du tahitien contemporain.* Paris: O.R.S.T.O.M.

Levy, Robert
   1967   Tahitian Folk Psychotherapy. *International Health Research Newsletter* 9:12–15.
   1973   *Tahitians: Mind and Experience in the Society Islands.* Chicago: University of Chicago Press.

Lewis, Nancy
   1981   Ciguatera, Health and Human Adaptation in the Island Pacific. Ph.D. diss., University of California, Berkeley.

Lieban, Richard W.
   1973   Medical Anthropology. In *Handbook of Social and Cultural Anthropology*, ed. John Honigmann, 1031–1072. Chicago: Rand McNally and Co.

Ludvigson, Tomas
   1981   Kleva: Some Healers in Central Espiritu Santo, Vanuatu. Ph.D. diss., University of Auckland.

Macdonald, Barrie
   1975   Secession in the Defence of Identity: The Making of Tuvalu. *Pacific Viewpoint* 16:26–44.
   1982   *Cinderellas of the Empire: Towards a History of Kiribati and Tuvalu.* Canberra: Australian National University Press.

Macdonald, Christine
   1973   *Medicines of the Maori.* Auckland: William Collins, Ltd.

MacKenzie, Margaret
   1973   Sociocultural Aspects of Preschool Child Health: Rarotonga, Cook Islands. Ph.D. diss., University of Chicago.

Macrae, Sheila
   1980   "Mortality" and "Fertility." In *A Report on the Results of the Census of the Population of Tuvalu, 1979,* ed. S. Iosia, S. Macrae, E. Bailey, and K. Groenewegen, 42–49, 33–41. Funafuti, Tuvalu: Government of Tuvalu.

Martin, John, ed.
   1827   *An Account of the Natives of the Tonga Islands in the South Pacific Ocean.* Edinburgh: Constable and Co.

Maude, H.
   1981   *Slavers in Paradise: The Peruvian Labour Trade in Polynesia, 1862–1864.* Canberra: Australian National University Press.

McArthur, Norma
   1967   *Island Populations of the Pacific.* Honolulu: University of Hawaii Press.

McHugh, Peter
   1968   *Defining the Situation.* Indianapolis, Ind.: Bobbs-Merrill Co.

Mead, Margaret
   1939   Native Languages as Field-work Tools: *American Anthropologist* 41:189–206.

Meleiseā, Penelope
   1979   Daughters of Sina: A Study of Gender, Status and Power in Western Samoa. Ph.D. diss., Australian National University.

Metge, Joan
   1978   *The Maoris of New Zealand.* 2nd ed. Boston and London: Routledge and Kegan Paul.

Milner, George
   1978   *Samoan Dictionary.* Interim ed. Manila: Samoa Free Press.

Morrison, James
   1935   *The Journal of James Morrison, Boatswain's Mate of the Bounty.* Ed. Owen Rutter. London: Golden Cockerel Press.

Munro, Doug
   1980   Tom De Wolf's Pacific Adventure: The Life History of a Commercial Enterprise in Samoa. *Pacific Studies* 3 (2): 22–40.

Nadeaud, J.
   1873   *Énumération des plantes indigènes de l'ile de Tahiti.* Paris: Libraire de la Société Botanique de France.

Neich, L., and R. Neich
   1974   Some Modern Samoan Beliefs Concerning Pregnancy, Birth and Infancy. *Journal of the Polynesian Society* 83 (4): 461–65.

New Zealand Department of Statistics
   1971   *New Zealand Census of Population and Dwellings.* Wellington: Government Printer.
   1976   *New Zealand Census of Population and Dwellings.* Wellington: Government Printer.

Noricks, Jay
   1981   The Meaning of Niutao *Fakavalevale* (Crazy) Behaviour: A Polynesian Theory of Mental Disorder. *Pacific Studies* 5:19–33.

Oliver, Douglas
   1974   *Ancient Tahitian Society.* 3 vols. Honolulu: University of Hawaii Press.

Oppenheim, Roger
   1973   *Maori Death Customs.* Auckland: A. H. and A. W. Reed Ltd.

Panoff, Michel
   1966   Recettes de la pharmacopée tahitienne traditionelle. *Journal d'Agriculture Tropicale et de Botanique Appliquée* 13:619–40.

Papy, Rene
   1954–   *Tahiti et les iles voisines.* 2 vols. Travaux du Laboratoire Forestier de
   1955   Toulouse. Toulouse: Douladoure.

Parham, B. E. V.
   1972   *Plants of Samoa.* Wellington: Government Printer.

Parham, H.
   1943   *Fiji Native Plants and Their Medicinal and Other Uses.* Memoirs of the Polynesian Society no. 16. New Plymouth, New Zealand: The Polynesian Society.

Parsons, Claire D. F.
   1978   The Health Care Process of a Rural Maori Population: The Ngāti Kahungunu Tribe of Wairoa. Department of Community Health, School of Medicine, University of Auckland.
   1981a   Sickness Experience and Language: Aspects of Tongan and Western Accounting. Vol. 1. Ph.D. diss., Waikato University.
   1981b   Sickness Experience and Language: Aspects of Tongan and Western Accounting. Vol. 2. Ph.D. diss., Waikato University.
   1981c   Tongan Sickness Conditions and Their Therapies. Glass Case, New Zealand and Pacific Collection, University of Auckland Library.

1983   Developments in the Role of the Tongan Healer. *Journal of the Polynesian Society* 92 (1): 31–50.

1984   Idioms of Distress: Kinship and Sickness Among the People of the Kingdom of Tonga. *Culture, Medicine and Psychiatry* 8 (1): 71–93.

Pearse, A.
1878   Letter to the L.M.S. from Raiatea, Society Islands, dated January 28. LMS South Seas Letters. Microfilm, Alexander Turnbull Library, Wellington.

Petard, Paul
1948   Description et usages de quelques plantes indigènes de Tahiti. *Journal de la Société des Océanistes* 4:115–31.

1972   *Raau Tahiti. Plantes médicinales polynésiennes et remèdes tahitiens.* South Pacific Commission Technical Document no. 167. Noumea: South Pacific Commission.

Powell, Thomas
1886   *O Le Tala I Tino O Tagata Ma Mea Ola Ese'Ese.* London: Unwin Brothers, The Gresham Press.

Prior, Ian
1971   The Price of Civilization. *Nutrition Today* 6 (4): 2–11.

Prior, Ian et al.
1966   *The Health of Two Groups of Cook Island Maoris.* Department of Health, Special Report. Series no. 26. Wellington: Medical Research Council of New Zealand.

Rosengren, Karl Erik
1976   Malinowski's Magic: The Riddle of the Empty Cell. *Current Anthropology* 17:667–85.

"R.V."
1925   Le guérisseur indigène à Tahiti. *L'Anthropologie* 35:197–98.

St. John, Harold, and Albert C. Smith
1971   The Vascular Plants of the Horne and Wallis Islands. *Pacific Science* 25 (3): 313–48.

Salmon, J.
1955   L'utilisation populaire des plantes médicinales à Tahiti. *Journal d'Agriculture Tropicale et de Botanique Appliquée* 2:438–42.

Sasportas, L.
1924   Le guérisseur indigène à Tahiti. *Aesculape* 14:237–41.

Savage, Stephen
1962   *A Dictionary of the Maori Language of Rarotonga.* Wellington: Department of Island Territories.

Schoeffel, Penelope
1980   Daughters of Sina. Ph.D. diss., Australian National University.

References

Schwartz, Lola
　1969　The Hierarchy of Resort in Curative Practices: The Admiralty Islands, Melanesia. *Journal of Health and Social Behavior* 10:201–209.

Shore, Bradd
　1977　Social Order and Social Control in a Polynesian Paradox. Ph.D. diss., University of Chicago.

Solomon Islands Statistics Division
　1980　*Report on the Census of Population 1976*. Honiara: Ministry of Finance.

Spillius, James
　1957　Polynesian Experiment: Tikopian Islanders as Plantation Labour. *Progress* 46 (256): 91–96.

Stair, J. B.
　1897　*Old Samoa, or Flotsam and Jetsam etc.* London: The Religious Tract Society.

Turner, George
　1861　*Nineteen Years in Polynesia*. London: Macmillan.
　1884　*Samoa a Hundred Years Ago and Long Before*. London: Macmillan.

Tuvalu Language Board
　1980　Tuvalu Language Board Recommendations on Orthography and Syntax; Policy 01/80. 20 August 1980. Funafuti: Tuvalu Language Board.

Tyrrell, D.
　1977　Aspects of Infection in Isolated Communities. In *Health and Disease in Tribal Societies*. Ciba Foundation Symposium 49. New series. Amsterdam: Elsevier Excerpta Medica.

Vayda, Peter
　1958　The Pukapukans on Nassau Island. *Journal of the Polynesian Society* 67:256–65.
　1961　Love in Polynesian Atolls. *Man* 61:204–205.

Vegan Welfare and Communication Centre of New Zealand
　n.d.　*Maori Medicine*.

Venner, Robert
　1944　Filarial Problem on Nanumea. *Naval Medical Bulletin* 43 (5): 955–63.

Vivian, J.
　1871–　South Seas Journals. London Missionary Society Records Relating to
　1872　the South Seas, 1796–1899.

Walker, Orsmond
　1925　Tiurai le guérrisseur. *Bulletin de la Société d'Études Océaniennes* 1:1–35.

Wax, Murray, and Rosalie Wax
　1963　The Notion of Magic. *Current Anthropology* 4:495–518.

Weiner, Michael A.
   1971   Ethnomedicine in Tonga. *Economic Botany* 25: 423–50.

Western Pacific High Commission
   1909   Secretariat, Inwards Correspondence, General: Minute Paper 289/1909. Records now held at Public Records Office, London.

Wilkes, C.
   1845   *Narrative of the U.S. Exploring Expedition During the Years 1838, 1839, 1840, 1841, 1842.* Philadelphia: Lea and Blanchard.

Wilson, John
   1978   Tuvalu Achieves Independence. *Commonwealth Law Bulletin* 4 (4): 1003–1009.

Winch, Peter
   1964   Understanding a Primitive Society. *American Philosophical Quarterly* 1:307–24.

Winkleman, Michael
   1982   Magic: A Theoretical Reassessment. *Current Anthropology* 23:37–66.

World Health Organization
   1966   *The Midwife in Maternity Care. Report of a W.H.O. Expert Committee.* WHO Technical Report Series 33.
   1978   *The Promotion and Development of Traditional Medicine.* WHO Technical Report Series 622.

Index

Animals, 162
Attack (*see also* Spirit sickness): of soul by spirits, 77; by spirits, 95, 106 n.6, 118, 142
Axes. *See* Red hot axes

Blood: bad blood, 39, 152; health, "enough blood" for, 152; spirit stepping on, 54
Bloodletting. *See* Treatments
Burial of dead, 131

Children: and medicines' effectiveness, 137–38; souls acquired from God, 165; vulnerability to soul loss, 77; vulnerability to spirits, 54, 142, 151
Christianity: influence on sickness explanation, 3–4, 51, 84, 131; influence on therapy, 29
Coconut oil: anointing with, 42, 209; spitting of, by healer, 42; treatments using, 18, 32, 37, 38, 40, 41, 42, 43, 48 n.11, 49 n.18, 80, 106 n.9, 154, 157, 225
Confession and Forgiveness: of misbehavior (clients'), 12, 61, 69, 79, 140, 143, 151; of misbehavior (family members'), 12, 61, 69, 148, 151, 159; as therapy, 12–13, 69, 140
Counseling, 228
Curing, experimentation in, 10, 135, 202
Cursing, 8, 78, 81–82, 141–42

Diagnosis (*see also* Dreams; Massage: in diagnosis): categories and procedure of, 11–13, 23, 51–57, 70–78, 85, 91–100, 117, 134–36, 138, 139, 140–41, 148–50, 153–55, 161–79; crabs used in, 231; limes used in, 171; of spirit possession, 95, 118, 119–20, 132, 139–40, 170–79; as western classification, 62, 100–101
Dispensaries, 32–33, 161
Dreams, 131–32, 154; causing sickness, 118–19, 149; diagnostic, 40, 81, 132; erotic, 178; predicting sickness, 27, 81; soul leaving the body during, 77, 165

Emotions causing illness: anger, 55, 64, 142; distress, 140, 141, 143; fanaticism or devotion, 140; fear, 149, 221; guilt, 140, 217; sexual arousal, 55
Exhumation, 98–99, 106 n.8

Faith healers, 228
Family: diagnoses, 135, 167; gods, 8, 151; sicknesses, 81, 99; spirits, 35, 132, 166; support of, during illness, 44–45, 143, 167
Family planning, 31, 76, 206
Food: and health, 152, 164; hot and cold foods, 134, 136; and illness, 54–55, 151, 152, 153, 164; and obesity, 152; and spirits, 54; *tapu* or restrictions on, 60, 134, 136, 152 (*see also* Prohibitions and *tapu*s)

Ghost sickness. *See* Spirit sickness
Gift of healing. *See* Power
Gifts: to gods, 8; to healers, 10, 132, 143, 154, 170–71, 204, 228

Hawaiians in Samoa, 5
Healers: attributes of, 10, 153; of broken bones, dislocations, sprains, 10, 72, 96; *faito'o* (Tonga), 90; *finematu'a* (Futuna), 113; gender of, 9, 10, 36, 72, 113, 114, 153–54, 168, 221, 228; *kleva* and *dresa*

(Vanuatu), 57; referrals of clients, 6–7, 11, 12, 97; relative as, preference for, 36, 59; respect for, 43, 72, 96, 132, 143, 154, 181, 203, 213, 216, 230; restrictions on during therapy, 43 (*see also* Food; Prohibitions and *tapu*s); risks of, 43; of skin and internal illnesses, 10, 97; *tahu'a* (Tahiti), 168, 173, 176–79; *taulasea* and *taula-aitu*, as *fofo* (Western Samoa), 5–6, 9; *ta'unga* (Rarotonga), 131; *tohunga* (New Zealand Maori), 213, 233; *tufunga* and *tino fai vai* (Tuvalu), 24, 35–36, 42–44

Healing practices: gaining knowledge of, 10, 202; of lay community members, 9, 58, 113, 114, 167, 168–71 (*see also* Lay understanding); specialization of, 11, 168

Healing practices, indigenous
—indigenous evaluations of, x; New Zealand Maori, 216, 233; Pukapuka, 153, 155; Rarotonga, 131, 143; Tahiti, 171, 181; Tikopia, 85; Tonga, 89–90, 92; Tuvalu, 46; Western Samoa, 1, 6, 203
—modification of, 6, 160
—origins, explanation of, 6
—prohibition of, 30, 84, 89, 213

Health, indigenous views of (*see also* Food; Blood): Futuna, 116, 121; New Zealand Maori, 215–16, 221, 224; Pukapuka, 144, 152, 155; Tahiti, 163, 166–67; Tikopia, 69, 70, 77; Tonga, 89–91; Tuvalu, 44

Heat application. *See* Treatments

Herbal plants, exotic: Western Samoa, 4; Tuvalu, 35, 36–37; Futuna, 110, 121; New Zealand Maori, 224

Herbal remedies: Futuna, 112–16, 119, 123–28; New Zealand Maori, 222–24, 225, 226, 227–28; Rarotonga, 136–38; Tahiti, 168–79, 185–98; Tikopia, 72; Tonga, 103–105; Tuvalu, 34, 35, 36–37; Vanuatu, 57–58; and weather, 138 (*see also* Moon; Weather); Western Samoa, 8–9

Hospitals: indigenous attitudes toward, 31–32, 91, 93, 135, 161, 218–20; and violation of *tapu*, 219

Hot and cold illnesses (*see also* Illness), 134

Hot and cold medicines (*see also* Treatment), 134, 136, 138; and moon, 137–38

Illness. *See also* Diagnosis
—contact and influenza epidemics, 2, 73, 84, 106 n.1

—contact with foreigners: New Zealand Maori, 213; Pukapuka, 146–51; Tikopia, 68, 73–74, 84; Tonga, 106 n.1; Tuvalu, 22, 47 n.6; Western Samoa, 2–4
—family susceptibility to, 29
—indigenous attitudes toward: Futuna, 121; New Zealand Maori, 215–16; Pukapuka, 155; Rarotonga, 143; Tahiti, 166–70; Tikopia, 69, 85; Tonga, 89–91, 92; Tuvalu, 44; Western Samoa, 203
—new illnesses, 90–100

Illness causation (indigenous), 28, 143
—biological or natural: Futuna, 117; New Zealand Maori, 217; Rarotonga, 133; Tahiti, 162, 171–73; Tikopia, 71; Tonga, 90, 96; Tuvalu, 25; Western Samoa, 2
—startlement or fright, 28
—supernatural: Futuna, 116–17; New Zealand Maori, 217–18; Pukapuka, 148–50; Rarotonga, 131–34; Tahiti, 164–66; Tikopia, 70, 77, 78; Tonga, 90–91, 94–95, 96; Tuvalu, 23–24; Vanuatu, 53–54; Western Samoa, 2, 3
—wrong naming, of children, 143

Infanticide: Tuvalu, 21; Western Samoa, 209–10

Injections, reactions to, 83, 91, 121

Kava, 56

Lay understanding: of western sickness explanations, 7, 34, 155; of western therapies for supernaturally caused illnesses, 34, 91–92, 131, 135, 136, 143, 155, 181

Magic: fishing magic, 27; growing magic, 58; love magic, 28, 35, 58; misuse of, 26, 49 n.11; sorcery, 58 (*see also* Sorcery); spells, 26, 40; Tuvalu, 26, 40, 48, 49 n.11; Vanuatu, 58–60; weather magic, 58

Mana. See Power

Massage, 34, 35, 112; aggravating illness, 135; application in healing, 98, 104, 119, 148, 153, 154, 204, 206, 207–208, 210, 225, 226; in diagnosis, 148, 153, 156, 204; types, 8, 38–39, 72, 101–103, 113–14, 138–39

Masseurs, 8, 138, 139

Medicine. *See* Healers; Healing practices; Herbal remedies; Treatments

Mental illness (*see also* Sorcery; Spirit sickness), 81, 95, 129, 140, 216, 217; explanations of, by Christian Church, 29; and full moon, 29

Index

Midwives: *fa'atosaga*, 201, 202; massage, use of, 38; respect for midwives, 200; Traditional Birth Attendants (TBA's), 201
Missionaries (*see also* Christianity; Pastors and priests): accounts of traditional treatments, 8, 29, 94, 131, 158–60; herbal remedies, use of, 4; own health, 3, 149; regard for healers, 43, 158–60; Samoan translations, 4; treating illness, lack of success in, 3–4
Moon: medicines affected by, 137, 138; spirits affected by, 131; tides affecting illness, 172; and treatment of mental illness, 29

Obesity, 152

Passion. *See* Emotions causing illness
Pastors and priests (*see also* Christianity; Missionaries): role as health advisor, 221; Samoan pastors, 4; status as healers, 216
Placenta, burial of, 209, 226–27; umbilical cord, burial of, 219
Power
—as *mana*, 69, 132, 137, 141
—of pastors and priests to heal, 80, 216
—of Samoan pastors in Tuvalu, 19
—spiritual, of healer, 25, 43, 132, 175–76
—supernatural: to attain goals, 24, 35; causing sickness, 39; of gods, 8, 148–50; to harm, 24, 36, 43, 48, 49, 55–57, 69, 77, 82–83, 131, 132, 136, 140; to heal, 24, 36, 69, 83, 132, 136, 213; to heal as gift of God, 9, 43, 132, 202
—therapies, 40–44, 49 n.14
Prayer: and healing, 43, 78, 80, 82, 83, 102, 113, 121, 213, 218, 221, 230–32; to ward off spirits, 217; and water, to lift *tapu*, 221, 232 (*see also* Prohibitions and *tapu*s)
Pregnancy (*see also* Prohibitions and *tapu*s: during pregnancy): postnatal complications, 211; seen as sickness, 203, 205
Pressure application. *See* Treatments
Prohibitions and *tapu*s: breaking of, 26, 30, 133–34, 136, 151, 152, 163, 217; on eating fish, 152; on intercourse in postnatal period, 210; during pregnancy, 30, 90, 106 n.3, 205; on whistling, 95
Psychic healers, 228

Red hot axes, in diagnosis and treatment, 16, 41–42, 43, 49 n.16
Ringatū penny, 229, 233, 234 n.8

Sneezing, 77
Sorcery: in court cases, 41; and healers, 41; Tikopia, 81; Tuvalu, 25, 36, 39, 40–44, 49; Vanuatu, 53, 55–57
Souls. *See* Spirits
Soul stealing, 54, 56
Spells (*see also* Magic), 26, 39, 40, 41, 42, 49 n.18, 81, 102
Spirit mediums, or familiars (*see also* Dreams): Rarotonga, 131, 132, 137, 139, 140; Tahiti, 158, 175, 177, 178; Tikopia, 67, 78, 80, 82, 83; Western Samoa, 8
Spirits: affecting treatment, 138; ancestral, 35, 78, 84, 94, 144, 146, 148; attributes of, 26, 54, 95, 106 n.6, 131, 148, 165–66; behavior punished by, 28, 79–80, 95, 118, 131–34, 139, 142, 149, 166, 177–79, 180, 182, 205, 216–18; causing offense to, 2, 69, 78, 79–80, 139, 142, 148, 155, 216–18; clan spirits, 79, 80; family spirits, 12, 24, 54, 78, 90, 94, 118, 130, 137, 142, 146, 205; foreign spirits, 149–50; power of, 8, 35, 136, 137, 140 (*see also* Power); seeking diagnostic information from, 35, 82, 139; seeking protection from, 35; talking spirits, 53–54
Spirit sickness: Futuna, 113, 116–17, 118–20; as means of social control, 143, 182–83; New Zealand Maori, 216–18, 229–33; Pukapuka, 146, 148–50; Rarotonga, 130–34, 137, 138–43; spirit possession, 28–29, 78–82, 94–95, 118, 132, 136, 138–40, 177–79; susceptibility to, 29, 178; Tahiti, 159, 163–79; Tikopia, 77, 78, 80–82; Tonga, 90, 94–95, 104; Tuvalu, 24, 26–30, 40–44; Vanuatu, 53–54, 56–57, 59, 61; Western Samoa, 9, 12, 73
Startle or fright illness, 28
Street kids: abortives used by, 225, 226; alcohol and drug abuse, 224; pregnancy, 224–26
Supernatural illnesses (*see also* Spirit sickness): *aitu* (Tuvalu), 24; *aitu* (Western Samoa), 2–3; *āvaga* (Futuna), 116, 118–20; *āvanga* (Tonga), 90, 94–95; *mahaki māhei* (Tuvalu), 25, 48 n.11; *ma'i tūpāpa'u* (Tahiti), 164–66; *maki tūpāpaku* (Rarotonga), 133, 136; *mate Maori* (New Zealand Maori), 216
Support networks. *See* Family: support of, during illness
Surgical skills: idigenous, 30, 34, 121, 158; missionaries, taught by, 4; penile superincision, 122

Tapu. See Prohibitions and *tapu*s
Taulu, 94; *taula-aitu* (Western Samoa), 7–8, 12
Toddy, 26
Tongans: early Tongan healers in Samoa, 5; influence of, in Wallis and Futuna, 109
Traditional Medicine. *See* Healing practices, indigenous; Treatments
Treatment
—expectation of rapid cure from, 92, 113, 174
—range of: Futuna, 122, 123–28; New Zealand Maori, 220, 222–33; Pukapuka, 154–55; Rarotonga, 136–43; Tahiti, 167–98; Tikopia, 71–84; Tonga, 100–105; Tuvalu, 18–19, 34–44; Vanuatu, 57–64; Western Samoa, 11–13, 204–11
—spirits affecting treatment, 138
—taking multiple treatments, 80, 135
—taking western and indigenous treatments, 7, 32, 135
Treatments (*see also* Herbal remedies; Massage): bloodletting, 34, 49; exhumation, 98, 99; heat application, 34, 37; power therapies, 40–44; pressure application, 34, 38; red hot axe treatments, 16, 41–42; surgery, 34, 121, 122

Washing: prior to therapy, 44; to spiritually cleanse, 229, 233; to ward off spirits, 229
Water (*see also* Herbal remedies; Prayer: and water; Washing), 228–29, 233
Weather (*see also* Moon), 152, 153, 163–64
Western medicine, indigenous evaluations of: Futuna, 117, 121–22; New Zealand Maori, 221, 230, 233; Rarotonga, 136, 143; Tahiti, 160, 181; Tonga, 91–100, 105; Tuvalu, 30, 34, 46; Western Samoa, 6–7
Western Samoa: influence of German administration on, 5; modification of traditional healing practices of, 4, 6; women's committees, 201, 202, 203
World Health Organization, ix

Contributors

Josephine Baddeley received her M.A. and Ph.D. in anthropology from the University of Auckland. Her research has included fourteen months of fieldwork in Rarotonga, Cook Islands. She is currently a barrister in Auckland specializing in criminal and family law.

Bruce Biggs was Professor of Maori Studies and Oceanic Linguistics at the University of Auckland, where he received his training in anthropology. He trained in linguistics at Indiana University. He is a Fellow of the Royal Society of New Zealand and past President of the Polynesian Society. His books include *Maori Marriages, Let's Learn Maori,* and the *Complete English-Maori Dictionary.*

Anne Chambers teaches cultural anthropology at Southern Oregon State College, Ashland. She received her M.A. and Ph.D. in anthropology from the University of California, Berkeley. Her research has included twenty-seven months of fieldwork in Tuvalu in 1973–1975 and 1983–1984, focusing on social organization, economics, and health and reproduction on Nanumea atoll.

Keith Chambers is Director of International Programs and Adjunct Professor of Anthropology at Southern Oregon State College, Ashland. He received his M.A. and Ph.D. in anthropology at the University of California, Berkeley. His research includes work in the Marshall Islands and more than two years of fieldwork in Tuvalu, primarily on Nanumea atoll. Publications include articles on social organization, expressive culture, and European contacts in the Pacific.

Julia A. Hecht received her Ph.D. in anthropology from the University of Chicago and a Masters in Public Health from the University of Hawaii. Her research has focused on family and community organization in Pukapuka and on social support and stress in American Samoa.

She is now Senior Policy Analyst Programmer at the Center for Health Studies of the Group Health Cooperative of Puget Sound, Seattle, where her current research interests are in gerontological health and the costs and modalities of care of chronic medical conditions.

Antony Hooper is Professor Emeritus of Social Anthropology at the University of Auckland and a Fellow in the Pacific Islands Development Program at the East-West Center, Honolulu. He received his M.A. from the University of Auckland and a Ph.D. in anthropology from Harvard University. He has done field research in the Society Islands and Tokelau, as well as among Cook Islander migrants in Auckland.

Patricia Kinloch Laing received her Ph.D. in anthropology from the University of Wellington. Her research focused on Western Samoa and Samoan people in Wellington. Currently Senior Lecturer and Associate Dean (Research) in the Faculty of Arts at Victoria University of Wellington, she teaches and supervises postgraduate students in social work, social science research, and nursing. She has published in the areas of health and traditional healing in the South Pacific and recently edited a special issue of the journal *Sites* on qualitative health research in New Zealand.

Tomas Ludvigson received his Ph.D. in anthropology from the University of Auckland, where he currently teaches anthropology and supervises graduate and postgraduate research, often in medical anthropology. He has conducted fieldwork in Espiritu Santo, Vanuatu, including a recent visit on behalf of the South Pacific Biodiversity Conservation Program, and in Indonesia.

Judith Macdonald received her Ph.D. from the University of Auckland in anthropology. She is currently a lecturer at the University of Waikato in Hamilton, New Zealand. Her research and teaching interests are in the fields of health and gender.

Cluny Macpherson received his M.A. in social anthropology from the University of Auckland, and a Ph.D. in sociology from the University of Waikato. Currently Associate Professor and Head of the Department of Sociology at the University of Auckland, he is the author of numerous articles on Samoan migrants, the coauthor of *Emerging Pluralism: Samoan Migrants in Urban New Zealand* and *Samoan Medical Belief and Practice,* and coeditor of *Nga Take: Ethnicity and Racism in Aotearoa/New Zealand.*

Claire D. F. Parsons received her Ph.D. in sociology from the University of Waikato, New Zealand, and was Claude McCarthy Fellow and Postdoctoral Fellow in Medical Anthropology at Harvard University. In

1994 she was a National Health and Medical Research Fellow in Public Health, which allowed her to work with colleagues at the University of California–San Francisco, the University of Colorado, and McMaster University. Since 1990 she has been Director of Research at the Centre for Research in Public Health and Nursing, La Trobe University, Melbourne, where she is also Director of Australia's National Priority Program entitled "People Living with HIV/AIDS and Their Carers." She has conducted fieldwork in the Kingdom of Tonga and among the Maori people of New Zealand and currently undertakes international research and publishes mainly in the areas of cultural health care issues, women's health, and HIV/AIDS.